# Self-help for Trauma Therapists

For those offering trauma-informed care, it can be difficult to maintain well-being and a balanced, positive outlook when the nature of their job requires frequent engagement with traumatic disclosures. *Self-help for Trauma Therapists: A practitioner's guide* intends to assist human service workers – such as those working as therapists, social workers and counsellors – to maintain their self-care and professional effectiveness when working in fields where stress and trauma play a key role in their everyday working lives.

Adopting a comprehensive, multilayered approach to self-care, the book grounds its exploration of practice through researched accounts with experienced professionals. Including accounts from clinical psychologists, therapists, counsellors, social workers and the friends and family of people in these professions, this book creates a narrative on stress and trauma from the human service worker perspective. Interwoven with these stories of practice, the author includes reflections on her own experiences in practice over the past 25 years with trauma survivors. With discussions on risk and resilience, compassion fatigue and vicarious traumatization, readers are introduced to the theories and practical applications of developing a professional model for maintaining well-being and self-care in their work.

*Self-help for Trauma Therapists: A practitioner's guide* is the first book of its kind to be written solely for human service workers. It is essential reading for beginning and more advanced practitioners who are involved in working with trauma and recovery and will also be of interest to supporters of those working in the helping professions.

**Margaret Pack** is Associate Professor of Social Work and Deputy Head of School, Allied Health Australian Catholic University, Sydney, Australia. Her research interests include trauma and stress, theories of clinician self-care and social workers' theories for practice. She has a strong interest and training in Gestalt psychotherapy. She has worked in a national sexual abuse trauma centre with survivors of sexual abuse trauma as a specialist case manager. Her career has included practice as a mental health social worker, where she has developed new services and managed staff as a team leader. Originally from New Zealand, she has coordinated a national postgraduate programme at Victoria University of Wellington and led a team of social work academics at Charles Darwin University, Northern Territory.

# Self-help for Trauma Therapists

## A practitioner's guide

Margaret Pack

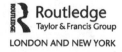

Routledge
Taylor & Francis Group

LONDON AND NEW YORK

First published 2017
by Routledge
2 Park Square, Milton Park, Abingdon, Oxon OX14 4RN

and by Routledge
711 Third Avenue, New York, NY 10017

*Routledge is an imprint of the Taylor and Francis Group, an informa business*

*British Library Cataloguing-in-Publication Data*
A catalogue record for this book is available from the British Library

*Library of Congress Cataloging in Publication Data*
Names: Pack, Margaret, 1961– , author.
Title: Self-help for trauma therapists : a practitioner's guide / Margaret Pack.
Description: Abingdon, Oxon ; New York, NY : Routledge, 2016. | Includes
bibliographical references and index.
Identifiers: LCCN 2016004014| ISBN 9781138898271 (hardback) | ISBN
9781138898288 (pbk.) | ISBN 9781315708676 (ebook)
Subjects: | MESH: Compassion Fatigue--psychology | Stress Disorders,
Traumatic--psychology | Self Care--methods | Social Workers--psychology |
Psychotherapy | Counseling
Classification: LCC RC552.P67 | NLM WM 172.4 | DDC 616.85/21--dc23
LC record available at http://lccn.loc.gov/2016004014

ISBN: 978-1-138-89827-1 (hbk)
ISBN: 978-1-138-89828-8 (pbk)
ISBN: 978-1-315-70867-6 (ebk)

Typeset in Times New Roman
by GreenGate Publishing Services, Tonbridge, Kent

For trauma therapists everywhere

In memory of my late Aunt, Janet Pack,
owner of 'Shrewberry' 1960–2005

# Contents

# Acknowledgements

Many friends and colleagues have contributed their time in the writing of this book. I am particularly grateful to the counsellor-participants and their friends, families and colleagues, who gave generously of their time to engage in in-depth interviews for the original research on which this book is based. Many of you have since become my friends and associates over subsequent years, adding insights to your original contributions to provide a longitudinal perspective.

I wish to acknowledge my debt to the founding work of the theorists who developed the vicarious traumatization framework including Dr Laurie Pearlman and the staff of the Traumatic Stress Institute; and Drs Judith Herman, Bessel van der Kolk and John Briere for their foundational theorizing about the 'new trauma therapy'; and Professor Charles Figley whose work collectively has assisted trauma therapists' efforts towards self-care internationally. Individually and collectively your work has greatly influenced my writing, and I deeply appreciate the many insights and contributions to our common enterprise. A special thanks goes to Professor Figley for agreeing to introduce the book through his foreword.

I also wish to thank my editorial assistant at Routledge, Louisa Vahtrick, Carrie Baker and Justin Cargill, of Victoria University, for assisting me in the editing process. Many thanks to Lianne Sherlock of Routledge, for designing the front cover from my photograph and an idea about self-care being a journey home. Special thanks to Dr Verna Schofield for assisting with final proofreading.

On behalf of Routledge, I wish to thank Taylor & Francis, SAGE, Gestalt Australia and New Zealand (GANZ), the New Zealand Association of Counsellors and Aotearoa New Zealand Association of Social Workers for generously allowing me to reproduce my previously published works over the last ten years (2004–2014).

On a personal note, I wish to thank my mother, Beryl Pack, and my sister, Robyn Pack, for their unerring support throughout the writing process. With such loyal and faithful support all things seem possible.

# Foreword

'I thought I made a big mistake the first time I sat alone in a room with a client.' It is a common reaction among new psychotherapists and others in direct practice working with the traumatized. Pioneer psychiatrist Lenore Terr's[1] first client was a young mother who abused her child and who herself was abused. Dr Terr had just had her first child and was now face-to-face with someone who regularly 'disciplined' her child but was never confronted because it wasn't done then. That was 1962. She went on to help create the modern field of trauma psychology. But it wasn't easy. She told me, and wrote in her autobiographical chapter, that images of abuse and flashbacks of clients reacting haunted her at times until she was able to figure out what was going on.

This book will help you figure out what's going on with you when certain clients trigger certain personal reactions; times when you are feeling exhilarated by the work followed by uncertainty, disgust, frustration, fear; being drawn to the work because it matters so much but repelled by its being so emotionally compelling and draining. And the book will guide you in developing an effective and sustainable self-care plan that takes into account your own personal experiences and needs, professional goals and life dreams.

It is noted towards the end of the book that the codes of ethics of many psychology, counselling, family therapy, social work, psychiatric and psychotherapy professional associations now incorporate standards of practice and ethical values; and codes of conduct expect practitioners to treat themselves, as needed, it being the responsibility of the practitioner to do the right thing, including sufficient attention to self-care. But this does not happen frequently. In most of my training sessions I ask the trainees, all practising professionals including psychotherapists, how many actually have a working self-care plan. 'It's in my head', is the common explanation when pressed. It is, therefore, unethical to practise with traumatized people without a specific self-care plan with appropriate indicators that at least one other person knows about. Otherwise, the quality of trauma-informed care will suffer because the impaired practitioner is not paying sufficient attention and applying sufficient emotional energy to their services.

Read this book and pass it on to a colleague who works with the traumatized. It may lessen your workload and increase your level of energy and it may do the same for your colleague.

Charles R. Figley, PhD
Paul Henry Kurzweg, MD Distinguished Chair in
Disaster Mental Health at Tulane University, New Orleans, USA
Editor, Routledge Psychosocial Stress Series

---

1  See Terr, L. (2006). Memoirs of a childhood trauma hunter. In C. R. Figley (Ed.), *Mapping trauma and its wake: Autobiographic essays by pioneer trauma scholars* (pp. 185–200). New York: Routledge.

# Preface

This book is written for all therapists who engage with traumatic disclosures from clients in the course of their work. In this chapter I introduce myself as author, and review some of the experiences that have been influential in the development of my interest in the impact of work as a trauma therapist.

I use the term *therapists* widely to include all those helping professionals who are involved in providing therapeutic services to survivors of trauma. In this way, I use the term therapist to refer to psychotherapists, clinical psychologists, social workers, mental health professionals and counsellors who deal with psychological trauma and its aftermath. This book aims to provide a self-care guide for those practitioners who engage empathetically with abuse survivors on a daily basis and in this process risk themselves becoming impacted by the nature of trauma-related contact. It is also a book about how trauma therapists and those in their social and professional networks actively evolve protective strategies and ways of being that enable them to remain effective professionals on the job. The approach the book takes is eclectic in that it aims to address the issues that face individual therapists and the wider structures that surround them. Drawing from a wide range of trauma theories is useful when dealing with traumatic disclosures as a therapist to form a unique framework for one's practice. Narrative, psychodynamic, gestalt, anti-oppressive and ecological systems approaches as well as trauma-informed theory are among those theories recommended to be a part of the therapist's essential repertoire of resources for understanding the complexity of working with trauma (Harms, 2015; Pack, 2014).

The inadequacy of language to express the unspeakable has meant that those who work with trauma and the traumatized face risks to their well-being through empathetic engagement with their clients. Actions, feelings, events and relationships can become alternative modes of expression beyond the verbal narratives of experience. Therefore, attending to what is happening in the individual therapist's relationships, world view and value base is insightful for how trauma-related work is impacting on their lives as it is suggestive of the ways in which the self of the therapist is being dynamically transformed (Pearlman and Saakvitne, 1996). To illustrate, I begin with a personal account of such transformative experiences in my professional life. These experiences set me on the path to wanting to write about the importance of the broader social contexts in trauma therapy, which are less prominent in the original vicarious traumatization framework described by McCann and Pearlman (1990). These experiences have sparked my lifelong interest in research on the various factors buffering these negative effects and the protective strategies evolved by trauma therapists.

# How this book came to be

Three sets of experiences within my own biography set me on the path of wanting to investigate the stress and trauma associated with working intensively with traumatic material from clients. The first of these formative events occurred in my first years of being a social worker in a mental health clinic, where the clients I was seeing disclosed details of early trauma histories when I was gathering routine personal background as part of an initial mental health assessment.

The second set of experiences occurred when I was working in a national trauma centre while researching my doctoral studies on vicarious traumatization among sexual abuse therapists. The third set of formative experiences coalesced when I was attending two psychotherapy conferences during the course of my training to become a psychotherapist. In these two conferences, for the first time I heard therapists talking openly about their experiences of being affected by the nature of their work and also the self-care strategies they were actively evolving to cope with the ongoing nature of the work. Rather than deal with the experiences chronologically, I begin with the most influential of these experiences.

At the time of researching and writing my PhD in the late 1990s, I was working as a case manager in a specialist national sexual abuse unit. In that role I was hearing and engaging on a daily basis with the graphic accounts of abuse and neglect from clients, and in this witnessing, gathering awareness of how deeply and irreversibly trauma transforms clients' lives. The secondary and vicarious impact of hearing these accounts of traumatic events was evident when recollections of client material weighed heavily on my mind long after the work day was over. I was aware of how my own values and beliefs were becoming affected. For example, there were parts of the country in which I was born and raised that no longer seemed safe to me when I witnessed survivor accounts from so many men, women and children who had been abused within these geographic locations. My home and sense of 'safe place' were irreversibly shaken. Taken-for-granted meanings of childhood being a time of innocence and relative emotional safety were similarly challenged. The widespread nature of abuse across the domains of class, gender, ethnicity and age became startlingly evident to me. The therapists who documented the various traumas and abuses in the reports I was daily reading to reach decisions about eligibility for treatment, I realized, were likely to be similarly impacted. While my role was to make judgements about the eligibility for the cover of claims for treatment and other costs, I was aware that there were emotional repercussions for the case managers and assessing therapists that were unacknowledged by the organizational structure at that time in the mid-1990s. Difficulties with staff morale, recruitment and retention persisted despite changes in personnel to the roles within the trauma unit. These events prompted a search for solutions in which I participated as an employee, enrolling in doctoral studies on the strength of the conundrum of organizational instability that we were all facing. This search involved management employing a team of psychologists for individual and team debriefing which resulted in staff psychological assessment and relocation of some affected staff to other units, yet the problems with staff morale and retention continued despite management's best efforts to assist individuals and the teams that surrounded them. As one of the two remaining original staff following this process with colleagues, staff and managers relocated or made redundant, I had a personal sense of survivor-hood and, though I remained working a total of ten years in the unit, I carried on with the knowledge that management in organizations dealing with trauma have a range of responsibilities to staff who work intensively with traumatic material.

The second formative experience inspiring this book came earlier in my career as a mental health social worker in the mid-1980s. In this context, I saw many clients who were referred by their general practitioners with depression and anxiety who during the initial assessment spontaneously began to discuss abuse and other early life traumas. As a generalist social worker, supported by a multidisciplinary team for whom trauma and recovery was considered a new area of expertise, I felt ill-prepared to work therapeutically with a caseload largely consisting of adults disclosing early abuse histories. The context of sexual abuse counselling in the 1980s, at the time I was employed in a community mental health clinic, was grounded in the feminist and self-help movement. This theory of recovery for sexual abuse survivors was imported from the United States of America so was not contextualized to Australasia. Beginning with the seminal writing of Bass and Davis's (1988) self-help guide entitled *The Courage to Heal*, which as clinicians we followed, the suggested approach was to support and facilitate disclosure of the traumatic events to form a coherent narrative for the survivor. The advice from such publications as Bass and Davis's (1988) *The Courage to Heal* was that narrative disclosure and catharsis were the means of healing from traumatic events. This understanding was challenged in the 1990s with the inception of the 'new trauma therapy' and the work of such theorists as Herman (1992), Briere (1996) and van der Kolk *et al.* (1996), where the advice was to assist in the rebuilding of self-worth, skills and esteem to ensure safety prior to memory work (Herman, 1992, 2010). While the 'new trauma therapy' is no longer quite so new, its authors' theorizing continues to shape trauma therapy today with updated insights remaining on the cutting edge of trauma therapy and intervention (for example, see Briere and Scott, 2014). The vicarious traumatization literature has grown exponentially also in areas such as mindfulness practice and spirituality as a source of renewal for therapists dealing with trauma (for example, see Follette *et al.*, 2015).

A third influence foreshadowing my interest coalesced when I was attending two conferences: Protecting the Frontline in July 1998 and eight years later a family therapy conference in 2006 which preceded a gestalt therapy conference that I was attending as part of my training in gestalt psychotherapy.

The Protecting the Frontline workshop was sponsored by the Delphi Centre of Australia. The Delphi Centre's founders Susan Henry and Naomi Halpern drew inspiration from the Delphi in ancient Greece and founded the Delphi Centre in Melbourne in 1985 when the theoretical frameworks to assist trauma survivors were being actively developed. Their centre provided therapists with a meeting place based in a holistic philosophy and approach towards developing professional identity through opportunities for all therapists regardless of background discipline and training. With the Delphi Centre as a central point of reference in the counselling and psychotherapy community, therapists in Australasia were encouraged to share networks, knowledge, experiences, expertise and resources through membership and training opportunities. Organizing for overseas experts to visit to bring new knowledge to Australian therapists was one role the Delphi Centre assumed.

At the Protecting the Frontline workshop organised by the Delphi Centre at Westmead Hospital, Sydney, Australia, I had the great honour of meeting Dr Laurie Pearlman, who together with colleagues from the Traumatic Stress Institute of Connecticut, USA, had developed constructivist self-development theory on which the concept of vicarious traumatization is based. The premise of constructivist self-development theory is that individuals are actively engaged in constructing their own reality through the development of patterns of thinking or 'cognitive constructs' that are used to interpret day-to-day incidents (McCann and Pearlman, 1990: 137).

Dr Pearlman acknowledged to the audience of this workshop in Sydney, some of the limitations of this theoretical model she was presenting from her research, including in her critique the theory's individualized focus. For example, Dr Pearlman acknowledged the wider social frameworks such as gender and power issues that underpin sexual abuse and domestic violence. These limitations and critiques of the theories being presented, once voiced led to conversations within a small workshop group of which I was a part about the structural inequality of Aboriginal people and their treatment by white Australia, to which trauma therapists in Australia are also witness. An example was given by the groups about the resources given by the Australian government to build the Olympic Games Village in Homebush, a suburb of greater Sydney. The scale of building on the construction of facilities for the Olympic Games not far from Westmead Hospital, where the workshop was located, was in contrast to the level of public funding provided for use in local Aboriginal communities. For many therapists, the work of sexual abuse therapy also explores the social inequality that surrounds trauma and issues of power in abuse and domestic violence. While there was some reference to the notion of connection to community in the vicarious traumatization literature, the theory behind it (constructivist self-development theory) seemed to me to be much grounded in the concepts and language of individual psychology.

The second time the issue of vicarious traumatization was raised for me was when I attended a family therapy conference in 2006 in Melbourne, Australia, when I was completing training in gestalt psychotherapy. The roundtable of keynote speakers was asked for their thoughts on how they were dealing with the stresses of being a psychotherapist working with survivor-related issues, including how they dealt individually with hearing traumatic disclosures from clients in the course of their work. Having completed my research with trauma therapists some years earlier, the comments from the panellists strongly resonated with my research findings that trauma therapists, through changing their relationships and networks, drew strength from their significant others to continue to work in this challenging field (Pack, 2004, 2009, 2014). The social, cultural, lifestyle and political aspects of the individual living in society were paramount to the participants I had interviewed for my research, which enabled them to balance hope for their clients in the face of client despair. This balancing of individual and structural analysis about the nature of sexual abuse recovery in society enabled them to remain fresh in their work to avoid burning out and becoming vicariously traumatized (Pack, 2004, 2009, 2014).

These experiences, therefore, began and furthered my thinking about the need to begin to investigate how therapists across a range of helping professions navigated the manifold impacts and effects of trauma-related work. In 2000 following ethical approval of my research proposal by the university in which I was studying, I interviewed 22 trauma therapists drawn from the national register of trauma therapists in New Zealand for my PhD research (Pack, 2004). Using semi-structured interviews, I asked the therapists and their significant others about what the impact had been upon their lives from working with sexual abuse disclosure during the course of their work. To add a further perspective, I interviewed separately the family members, friends, colleagues and supervisors who were nominated by the primary therapists. I asked the personal and professional significant others to comment upon what they had observed of changes in the therapist in a number of different areas of life, over the time in which they had known them. Through the therapists' own accounts of their experiences interwoven with the perceptions of their significant others, I identified a gap in the existing literature on the impact on therapists from their work in relation to the effects on the therapists' primary personal and professional relationships. While there were self-care workbooks on vicarious traumatization (Pearlman and Saakvitne, 1996) and social work guides (van Heugten, 2011), there was no self-care guide that I could locate that included the insights of significant others to add to the awareness of the therapist of their own process in relation to their significant relationships. I discovered that the partners, husbands, wives, adult children, colleagues and supervisors all had perceptive and incisive comments as to how their relationships with their loved ones and colleagues were transformed by the nature of the work in trauma care. This mirror image provided by the insights of the personal and professional others surrounding the therapist was a potent reminder of the changes in the therapist's sense of self over time, alerting them to the need to self-assess regularly as to what was happening in their own process.

This book aims to bridge this gap in the existing literature on vicarious traumatization to evolve understandings of the impact of trauma-related therapy drawing from both the insights of experienced trauma therapists and their significant others. To do this depth assessment I felt the need to update my original literature review to reflect the new theorizing about vicarious traumatization and related concepts, and to relate this to what the counsellor-participants continued to tell me over the years. These insights and resources are included at the end of each chapter, sometimes with personal recommendations from the counsellors who were interviewed.

## The structure of this book and how to approach its reading

I suggest that readers approach this book chapter by chapter reading only as little or much as they feel is helpful to illuminating their own process and themes. Some parts might be relevant, others less so, so I invite readers to use their discernment as to which parts apply to their experience. Questions for reflections, activities and a range of resources such as web links, reference lists and case studies are offered at the conclusion of each chapter and are to be referred to when a theme or issue resonates. The case studies within and at the conclusion of chapters are drawn from the therapists who participated in my research on vicarious traumatization. As agreed in the informed consent required as part of the research ethical approval, each participant is identified by the original pseudonyms they chose to represent their contribution. Each participant said that they wished to contribute to the research to illuminate a common experience. Where relevant and to illuminate themes, I frame the chapter with a quotation from one of the counsellor-participants or one of the conference keynote speakers in the roundtable preceding the Gestalt Psychotherapy Conference in 2008. Sometimes it can be reassuring to hear the stories of another within which we can resonate and develop our own stories and responses. Therefore, excerpts from other therapists and my own reflections about my own practice are offered to illustrate a theme or common experience.

As with all research, the starting point is to define and review the relevance of concepts and literature in relation to vicarious traumatization and therapist resilience with implications for self-care. Therefore, this is where I will begin in the first chapter. Chapter 2 introduces a multilayered model of stress and trauma based in my research with trauma therapists in the New Zealand context. This model enables us to see that vicarious traumatization can be viewed more systemically as a useful albeit challenging experience and as a phase in career that, successfully navigated, can develop personal resources for promoting professional effectiveness. The key theme is to address vicarious traumatization through self-care at a number of levels involving the self of the therapist, one's relationships, personal and professional, within one's employing organization, and tackling the societal discourses that surround trauma therapy and the work of recovery.

Chapter 3 outlines one of the major themes of Chapter 2 in that symptom-focused approaches lack the integrative and holistic healing potential of narrative to ameliorate vicarious traumatization for trauma therapists. This chapter suggests that awareness of one's personal and professional narratives, and the use of 're-authoring' (White, 1997), is a potent tool towards therapist self-care. Chapter 4 focuses on how therapists' relationships can be transformed over time by the nature of the work. The manifold implications of this finding for maintaining and in some cases changing one's relationships, personal and professional, to align with changes in the therapist's world view and belief systems are explored. Chapter 5 deals with clinical supervision and the models of supervision that are supportive to therapist well-being when working intensively with trauma disclosures. Dealing with parallel processes in the therapeutic relationship and traumatic transference by using a relational model of clinical supervision separate from line supervision functions, is suggested. Chapter 6 continues this theme to explore what the organizational issues are in addressing the potential for vicarious traumatization to keep employees and teams safe on the job. Chapter 7 focuses on the organizational provision of critical incident stress management (CISM) programmes guided by a literature review about models found most helpful when dealing with trauma. Chapter 8, 'The search for self and the search beyond self', explains the role of spirituality, belonging in nature and in community to evolve new ways of being as a trauma therapist that are conducive to self-nurturance. The effects of a greater sense of connection to self and other ultimately benefits one's clients as the self of the therapist is more open and available to the other in the therapeutic contact (Pack, 2014). Spirituality has been found to be growing in importance in the therapist self-care literature recently, with a focus on the effectiveness of mindfulness and integrated mind–body practices to ameliorate the effects of the work (Follette *et al.*, 2015; Pack, 2014).

Chapter 9 looks at career and lifestyle adjustments that bring into alignment the transformations that are occurring for the trauma therapist's sense of self, over time. Balancing interests, caseload and case composition, and work and leisure balance are discussed in this chapter. In Chapter 10, the final chapter, the themes of each chapter are drawn together into the model earlier outlined with implications for therapist self-care on each level of a multi-level systemic approach to vicarious traumatization and therapist resilience.

As with all chapters, my own reflections about engaging with trauma disclosures and the impact of this work are woven into the fabric of what the therapists participating in this research discussed with me during in-depth interviews for the research about their experiences of vicarious traumatization. The insights of the focus group of four trauma therapists who met to analyse with me the emerging findings are also included in each chapter.

I refer to the therapists interviewed for the research undertaken as the *participant-counsellors*, and their family, friends and supporters who were interviewed as the *significant other participants* to distinguish their contributions. While the original research was completed in 2002, the counsellor-participants have remained in contact with me in various ways, ever since, some becoming close friends, colleagues and associates. Others continued contact with me by email and through social media particularly when I relocated to Australia in 2011, many continuing to send me some of the self-care resources I have included in the further reading and resource lists at the conclusion of each chapter. They told me that they wished to bring their knowledge to a wider audience to support their colleagues.

As key theorists have served to provide the counsellor-participants with a 'road map' for their work with trauma survivors, I have included the now classic work of trauma theorists such as Briere, Herman, and van der Kolk, McFarlane and Weisaeth, among others, as 'way showers' to 'what works'. I have then juxtaposed these classic works with more recent trauma frameworks and literature to show the development of new directions in theory building about the impact of the work and what buffers or ameliorates it. As I discovered that narrative theory has a key contribution to make in the counsellor-participants' healing from vicarious traumatization, I have included the classic theorizing and work of the late Michael

White and his colleagues from the Dulwich Centre in what builds resilience for therapists who deal with trauma (White, 1995, 1997). Some of the narratives contain material that can be distressing to read. I suggest pacing your reading and discussing with colleagues and supporters, should personal issues arise for you.

With this explanation setting the context for what is to come, I will turn in the next chapter to define core concepts and to outline the rationale and aims of my research with trauma therapists. I then turn to the methodology of my original research and discuss how and why I decided to focus on how the therapists interviewed dealt with trauma. These narratives are told through the counsellor-participants' own stories and those of their families, partners, colleagues and friends.

I hope you find this a useful resource and I wish you well with the development of your own self-care plan.

Dr Margaret Pack
Associate Professor of Social Work
Australian Catholic University, Sydney, Australia

## References

Bass, E. and Davis, L. (1988). *The courage to heal: A guide for women survivors of child sexual abuse.* New York: Harper & Row.

Briere, J. (1996). *Therapy for adults molested as children* (2nd edn). New York: Springer.

Briere, J. and Scott, C. (2014). *Principles of trauma therapy: A guide to symptoms, evaluation, and treatment* (2nd edn). Thousand Oaks, CA: SAGE.

Follette, V. M., Briere, J., Rozelle, D., Hopper, J. and Rome, D. I. (2015). *Mindfulness-oriented interventions for trauma: Integrating contemplative practices.* New York: Guilford.

Harms, L. (2015). *Understanding trauma and resilience.* London: Palgrave Macmillan.

Herman, J. (1992). *Trauma and recovery: The aftermath of violence – From domestic abuse to political terror.* New York: Basic Books.

Herman, J. (2010). *Trauma and recovery: The aftermath of violence – From domestic abuse to political terror* (2nd edn, reprint). London: Pandora.

McCann, I. L. and Pearlman, L. A. (1990). Vicarious traumatisation: A framework for understanding the psychological effects of working with victims. *Journal of Traumatic Stress, 3* (1), 131–49. doi: 10.1002/jts.2490030110

Pack, M. J. (2004). Sexual abuse counsellors' responses to stress and trauma: A social work perspective. *New Zealand Journal of Counselling, 25* (2), 1–17. Retrieved from www.nzac.org.nz/new_zealand_journal_of_counselling.cfm (accessed 16 March 2016)

Pack, M. J. (2009). The body as a site of knowing: Sexual abuse therapists' experiences of stress and trauma. *Women's Study Journal, 23* (2), 46–56. Retrieved from www.wsanz.org.nz (accessed 16 March 2016).

Pack, M. (2014). Vicarious resilience: A multilayered model of stress and trauma. *Affilia: Journal of Women and Social Work, 29* (1), 18–29. doi: 10.1177/0886109913510088

Pearlman, L. A. and Saakvitne, K. W. (1996). *Transforming the pain: A workbook on vicarious traumatization.* New York: W. W. Norton.

van der Kolk, B. A., McFarlane, A. C. and Weisaeth, L. (Eds). (1996). *Traumatic stress: The effects of overwhelming experience on mind, body, society.* New York: Guilford Press.

van Heugten, K. (2011). *Social work under pressure: How to overcome stress, fatigue and burnout in the workplace.* London: Jessica Kingsley.

White, M. (1995). *Re-authoring lives: Interviews and essays.* Adelaide: Dulwich Centre Publications.

White, M. (1997). *Narratives of therapists' lives.* Adelaide: Dulwich Centre Publications.

# Other resources for self-care

## Traumatic Stress Institute resources

Pearlman, L. (1995). Self-care for trauma therapists: Ameliorating vicarious traumatization. In B. H. Stamm (Ed.), *Secondary traumatic stress: Self-care issues for clinicians, researchers, and educators* (pp. 51–64). Lutherville, MD: Sidran Press.

Pearlman, L. A. and Saakvitne, K. W. (1995). *Trauma and the therapist: Countertransference and vicarious traumatization in psychotherapy with incest survivors*. New York: W. W. Norton.

Pearlman, L. A. and Saakvitne, K. W. (1996). *Transforming the pain: A workbook on vicarious traumatization*. New York: W. W. Norton.

Saakvitne, K. W., Tennen, H. and Affleck, G. (1998). Exploring thriving in the context of clinical trauma theory: Constructivist self development theory. *Journal of Social Issues*, *54* (2), 279–99. Retrieved from http://onlinelibrary.wiley.com/doi/10.1111/j.1540-4560.1998.tb01219.x/pdf (accessed 28 February 2016).

## Compassion fatigue

Figley, C. (2002). Compassion fatigue: Psychotherapists' chronic lack of self care. *Psychotherapy in Practice*, *58* (11), 1433–41. Published online in Wiley InterScience (www.interscience. wiley.com). doi: 10.1002/jclp.10090. Retrieved from www.researchgate.net/profile/CR_Figley/ publication/11053266_Compassion_fatigue_Psychotherapists%27_chronic_lack_of_self_care/ links/0912f50588e4bd67ba000000.pdf (accessed 28 February 2016).

Mathieu, F. (2012). *The compassion fatigue workbook: Creative tools for transforming compassion fatigue and vicarious traumatisation*. New York: Routledge.

van Dernoot Lipsky, L. and Burk, C. (2009). *Trauma stewardship: An everyday guide to caring for self while caring for others*. San Francisco, California: Berrett-Koehler.

## Professional development training: the Delphi Centre

Pioneers of trauma professional development in Australasia. The link below takes you to the training catalogue 1995–2015. The centre offers consultation services, resources, a library and newsletter:

http://delphicentre.com.au/professional-development-training

To receive updated information on forthcoming seminars and specialist resources an online form enables you to join the network at:

http://delphicentre.com.au/join-our-network

## GANZ Gestalt Australia and New Zealand

Information on membership, forthcoming events, journal/newsletter and professional development opportunities:

https://ganzwebsite.wordpress.com

# Abbreviations

| | |
|---|---|
| ACC | Accident Compensation Corporation of New Zealand |
| ANZATSA | Australian and New Zealand Association for the Treatment of Sexual Abuse |
| APA | American Psychological Association |
| CISD | critical incident stress debriefing |
| CISM | critical incident stress management |
| DSM | *Diagnostic and Statistical Manual of Mental Disorders* |
| EMDR | Eye Movement Desensitisation and Reprocessing (therapy) |
| GANZ | Gestalt Australia and New Zealand |
| ISSC | Integrated Services for Sensitive Claims |
| ISST | International Society for the Study of Trauma and Dissociation |
| NTT | new trauma therapy |
| ProQOL | professional quality of life scale |
| PTSD | post-traumatic stress disorder |
| TA | transactional analysis |
| TSM | traumatic states of mind |

# Chapter 1    **What are stress and trauma and how do they impact?**

## Introduction

I have undertaken personal therapy since I started this job [trauma therapy in a family therapy agency] because, contrary to what I thought, as I trained more and worked deeper with clients, my heart has not closed, it has actually become more and more empathetic. There would have been lots of issues of transference and countertransference through time that I needed to work with. So I did a lot more work about my personal abuse over a number of years … I feel confident in my ability to make a difference in my world. I do. Because I think that the method I come from or my personal way of being in the world is body, mind and spirit being connected.

*Rose, a counsellor-participant discussing her approach to working in the field of trauma with survivor clients and her approach to her own healing over her 30 year career as a therapist.*

Working with trauma survivors is rewarding. It is also fraught with contradictions and challenges. In this chapter, I discuss the various concepts used to explain the experiences that can arise in work with trauma survivors. In the literature I have reviewed and in discussion with therapists who work in the field of sexual abuse trauma and recovery, I discovered that the impact of the work as a trauma therapist varies from worker to worker and is also dependent on a range of personal and professional factors, including their particular caseload mix and organizational context. Rose's comments above illustrate the importance of holism and a mind–body integrated approach when working with trauma. Personal therapy to develop awareness of the impact of the work as the therapist in a continuous way was also important in maintaining therapeutic effectiveness and well-being. Awareness is sometimes very difficult to develop when we are riding the high seas of client emotions and trying to manage our own feelings and responses as we listen empathetically to clients. As Rose indicates, the depth at which we engage can be a further variable to consider in how we are affected by the nature of the work. This is where the concepts of vicarious traumatization and compassion fatigue can help us to assess what is occurring in our responses as we engage with trauma survivors on the job.

As a starting point, then let's begin to examine the terminology used to describe trauma and stress to enable conceptual clarity about the definition of the various terms.

## Stress

We often refer to 'being stressed' when our lives are out of balance or we feel overwhelmed with a combination of conflicting emotions, due to onerous duties or responsibilities. Such situations can lead us to such responses as feeling under pressure. In the research litera-ture, stress is understood in terms of the impact of particular sources of stress known as 'stressors', which singularly or together impact on individuals to produce certain effects. These effects include physical manifestations such as the 'fight and flight response', where we attempt to fend off or avoid any perceived threat to our survival or well-being. The 'fight and flight' response can manifest in such physical symptoms we can experience in the body as heart palpitations, increased perspiration and nausea among other symptoms. Psychological effects often include negative thinking, anxiety or worry and behavioural manifestations such as insomnia, irritability and anger outbursts when we relate to others. Over time the triggering of such responses can result in coping strategies such as avoid-ance and absenteeism in the workplace, and persistent ill health such as catching colds and flus repeatedly, as such tensions can trigger the release of hormones such as cortisol that over time can affect the immune system (van Heugten, 2011). Muscular tension can lead to back and other health problems when apparently there is no physical or medical cause for ongoing aches and pains.

Some sources of stress are positive and are, in fact, necessary to motivate and so can lead to satisfaction and fulfilment. Therefore, some sources of work stress can have a positive impact on our well-being. How we perceive events as being 'stressful' or 'pleasurable' will depend on factors such as previous experiences/responses, and may be tied to personality styles and resources. Equilibrium in one's work–life balance, altruism and variety in case-load are also considered important in balancing stress with work rewards and a sense of fulfilment in one's personal and professional life (Collins, 2007; Gibbons *et al.*, 2011). For example, Sophia, one of the trauma therapists interviewed for my research, explains what sustains her in her work, in an excerpt from an interview below:

> Sophia: My life is much more satisfying now. I'm in charge of it [laugh] which is one thing I really like. Not being married is really good. I really love having my own place. I love it when the kids are this age now because they can look after themselves a lot now. I've got lots of good friends. Life's a struggle financially somewhat being solo. But my life is good, very full.
>
> (Pack, 2014)

Feeling that we hold the locus of control over our life with autonomy to make our own choices and decisions, is part of what can help us deal positively with the multiple chal-lenges of juggling work and personal demands. Where the locus of control feels constantly with the other, or out of our control consistently, feelings of powerlessness can be experi-enced which can be a source of 'burnout' (van Heugten, 2011). This is a term that is often discussed alongside vicarious traumatization and compassion fatigue, but is seen as having some distinct features.

## Burnout

The process of 'burnout' also seemed relevant to the experience of trauma therapists I interviewed as the process of stress in their experiences seemed to arise insidiously from exposure to traumatic client narratives. However, I noted from my reading that 'burnout' was often referred to in a more general sense as a term used to describe the 'fit' between the individual's belief system and the organization's philosophy, aims and tasks (Grosch and Olsen, 1994; Leiter and Maslach, 1988).

'Burnout' is seen as encompassing a range of components, including emotional exhaustion, feelings of depersonalization and a sense of reduced accomplishments in one's work (Stamm, 2005). The organizational culture is often cited as a source of burnout, when socioeconomic factors lead to retrenchment and reduced services which make it extraordinarily difficult for ethical therapists to meet their personal and professional ethical standards of practice (Fulcher, 1988). For example, van Heugten discusses in her research among social workers the many difficult adaptations that workers make to their changing work contexts during organizational restructuring, often culminating in decisions to leave and set up in private or group practices (van Heugten, 2011). The experience of lacking control over the way one does one's work can be linked to burnout, therefore (van Heugten, 2011). Individual symptomatology of burnout can often be an indicator of what is happening in the wider organizational culture and economy, yet this is often a neglected area in the literature where the focus is on individual responses with little attention given to the surrounding organizational and societal context in which practice occurs (Harms, 2015).

Lack of clarity about one's work role coupled with conflicting responsibilities on the job and a lack of support are other factors that contribute to 'burnout' (Leiter and Maslach, 1988). For example, Audrey, who was one of the counsellor-participants in my research, describes stress caused within her work as a child therapist when she was responsible for assessing whether the child had been abused or not. Those who began practising as trauma therapists from the mid-1970s onwards lacked the support of developed theory on trauma and support from a knowledgeable workforce to do the work. The effects of trauma on children who were abused were lacking a coherent evidence base and, therefore, best efforts were experimental and of necessity, tentative. Those who took up the challenge of offering therapy and assessment services became authorities whom others turned to. This expert role was neither sought nor wished for. Addressing societal disbelief was another factor contributing to Audrey's experience. A sense of emerging collegial camaraderie developed in the course of what Audrey described as a 'baptism by fire'. Part of the 'stress/burnout' was dealing with the backlash in bringing abuse to the public's attention and the lack of systems to support her assessment of complex situations where children were at risk of abuse:

> Audrey: When I first started working people didn't believe it [sexual abuse] occurred and so you copped a lot of flak in bringing it to people's attention. So I think it was actually far more stressful than I had imagined and I never imagined, like, going to court or anything like that. And there were no systems! [rolls her eyes] So that was far more stressful.

## Reflective questions

- Do these descriptions of stress and burnout resonate with your own experiences?
- How so – in what ways are they relevant or do they apply to your experiences?
- Are there signs that give you advance warning that stress and burnout are operating in your personal/professional life currently?
- In the past? (Notice any patterns in physical sensations, thoughts and behaviours.)
- Notice and describe whether there was a trigger to these signs of stress/burnout.
- What was happening at that time in your life?
- What are your 'early warning' signs of being under stress/burnout?
- What do you do when you are experiencing such signs?

## Trauma

Psychotherapists, regardless of the context of their practice, encounter clients who disclose traumatic histories. But what is trauma? Furthermore, which experiences are considered 'traumatic' and why? Trauma has been linked to a 'history of repeated interpersonal victimisation that has impacted adversely on a person's mental and potentially physical and social health across their life span' (Wall and Quadara, 2014: 4). Typically those who experience or witness an event considered to be 'traumatic' experience the intense fear, helplessness or horror of the person who goes through that event (American Psychological Association [APA], 2013). If the re-experiencing of this fear of life-and-death proportions inspires traumatic transference in the therapeutic relationship between client and therapist, there are special kinds of clinical supervision that are recommended that I will go on to discuss in Chapter 5.

Secondary traumatic stress can be triggered by witnessing the distress of others in the aftermath of trauma (Herman, 2010). I have briefly outlined in the preface the nature of some of the potential responses to trauma for trauma therapists without giving those experiences labels or names. Each may be distinguished from the other once we explore the theory behind each term, which is considered helpful for gaining an awareness of how these concepts relate to oneself and one's own process of dealing with traumatic material recounted in the course of therapy. In fact, an understanding of each concept and awareness of one's intra-psychic process is considered a protective factor to unravelling the impact of trauma on the therapist who engages in it. Herman (1992) in her seminal work *Trauma and Recovery* likens the therapist's responses to this engagement with trauma as a 'contagion' that gives some idea of how we affect one another by the telling and retelling our stories that involve traumatic material and particularly material relating to the intentional harm inflicted by one human being on another. As each individual therapist reacts differently to immersion in traumatic disclosures due to personal biographies, past traumas, personal resources and the use of support networks, I begin by outlining some of the main signs and symptoms that alert therapists that the work in the trauma field may be negatively impacting. This impact may be a fleeting experience or one that comes and goes such as acute stress responses. Alternatively it may be more permanently transforming as described in the literature on 'vicarious traumatisation' (McCann and Pearlman, 1990).

While sexual abuse trauma is considered to have distinctive features as a form of trauma, many abuses and traumas are widespread and interlocking with physical, psychological, sexual abuse overlaid with neglect resulting in harm to clients and their families, often across several generations. Age, gender, culture and life stage are also variables, with the vast majority of victims being children and women who have been abused by male perpetrators (Wall and Quadara, 2014: 6). The interaction of complex social problems and cultural factors compounds the already complex nature of abuse and violence. In Australia, Aboriginal women and children are among those most victimized with repeated and ongoing trauma resulting from violence and the impact of intergenerational trauma brought about by colonization and separation from lands and cultural identity (Wall and Quadara, 2014: 12–14). In working with clients who have been multiply abused across generations, trauma therapists often deal with complex trauma presentations that transcend service boundaries and the resources of even the most able of therapists. Accessing multiple services in a brokering fashion may be outside the scope of most therapists' training, and such work can be overwhelming in its range, complexity and scope. Due to this complexity an ecological systems or person-in-environment approach is recommended for understanding victimization and recovery of abuse survivors. This approach involves working within the systems and subsystems surrounding the victim, including family and community in the dimensions of intervention. For example, Grauerholz (2000) writes of child sexual abuse interrelating with subsequent relationships in which adult survivors are re-abused, suggesting the need for intervention on multiple fronts to address factors in the social environments in which people live.

Coupled with this complexity is the co-morbidity for other conditions such as addictions, depression and anxiety, and other personality disorders that are considered to be functional in terms of the original abuse experience (Herman, 2010).

To understand secondary impacts for therapists, it is useful to review the impacts for the clients that flow on to affect therapists through the dynamic process of transference and countertransference. The changes to the definitions of post-traumatic stress disorder (PTSD) in the Diagnostic and Statistical Manual of Mental Disorders (DSM) demonstrate the growth in trauma as a field of practice and the increasing recognition of the secondary impacts on observers, practitioners and supporters (APA, 2013). This growth is evident in the recent extensions of the diagnosis of 'post-traumatic stress disorder' which is a feature of most trauma presentations.

## Post-traumatic stress disorder

PTSD is a psychiatric diagnosis defined in the DSM-5 classificatory system of psychiatric disorders as being related to situations in which the individual is confronted by events that involve an actual or perceived threat to life, or an event that seriously threatens the physical integrity of oneself or others (APA, 2013). If the client's post-trauma signs and symptoms such as insomnia, hypervigilance, and energy and appetite problems continue unabated for three months or longer, chronic PTSD is usually diagnosed.

Chronic PTSD is thought to be underpinned by a potentially irreversible set of conditions (APA, 2013) though exactly why some individuals are more prone to developing longer-term conditions after experiencing traumatic events in relation to PTSD remains unclear.

In the DSM-5, the definition of 'trauma' within the diagnosis of PTSD now includes the secondary effects of those who witness trauma. Secondary traumatic stress is a term that involves the witnesses' experiences of persistent or recurrent images or thoughts of the event disclosed or seen by them (APA, 2013). These distressing images and recollections may manifest as flashbacks, thoughts and perceptions of the event, which may arise over time, intruding into and colouring everyday life.

Wilson et al. (2001: 3) advocate an expansion of the diagnosis of PTSD to explain a range of trauma-related phenomena due to the complexity of how trauma impacts and manifests:

> Posttraumatic phenomena and their permutations are rich in their tapestry and are woven of thousands of threads whose fibers are spun from unique and sometimes exotic, secretive, horrific, and forbidden sources of discovery. Working clinically or in research settings with PTSD is a journey of puzzlement, curiosity, fascination and uncertainty.

It is, therefore, critical that, as therapists, we become familiar with the secondary impacts of engagement with survivors who are experiencing the many complex manifestations of past and current trauma where PTSD and complex PTSD likely features.

## Personal reflections on how traumatic disclosures impact

To illustrate how this secondary traumatization process works in practice, I offer the following reflection on my experience as a mental health practitioner where I was seeing many clients who disclosed traumatic histories. As I began engaging empathetically with clients as a mental health social worker and later as a psychotherapist employed in a national trauma unit, I began to notice a transformation in my own thinking, beliefs and my sense of being. I wondered if this was evidence of some repressed memory of trauma in my own personal history though I could not recall any such incident from my childhood. With the benefit of hindsight, I realize I was living out a secondary traumatization process that was fuelled by traumatic transference and countertransference (Herman, 2010).

Engagement with narratives of survivorhood from women who had endured the worst effects of physical, sexual, psychological and spiritual abuse had a profound impact upon my life. The nature of the work heightened my sense of personal vulnerability and control in the world. I believe it is no coincidence that during this intensive immersion in these narratives I decided to join a self-defence training class for women and avoided walking alone at night. In retrospect, I was over-identifying with client narratives. I was travelling a parallel path to the traumatized clients whose stories filled my days in the mental health clinic in which I was working as a therapist. This parallel process is a kind of secondary traumatization specific to helping professionals. Terms such as: 'compassion fatigue', 'secondary traumatic stress', 'vicarious traumatization' and 'burnout' all have connections to this experience.

## Secondary traumatization/secondary post-traumatic stress

At first glance, the concept of 'secondary traumatization' appeared helpful to understanding my and the counsellor-participants' various experiences. This literature suggests that therapists' own empathetic engagement with the client's traumatic material can impact on the therapist in a variety of ways, including emotionally, and may be noticeable as physical signs and cognitive patterns as we saw in my personal experience above.

Feeling 'distressed' and having breathing problems was one example of this theme. One of the counsellor-participants, Audrey, explains her shock and disbelief when a child client she was seeing for assessment was abducted. Audrey thought this was a direct experience of being traumatized herself on the job rather than one vicariously experienced:

> Audrey: From memory the main thing I thought was I hadn't so much had vicarious traumatization as having been traumatized from the horrible stuff people told me and being made anxious by family group conferences, courts, and those incidents I told you about where actual things happened that distressed me. Like the child being abducted. So I was thinking of another way of looking at it. That is there is trauma that happens to us on the job.
>
> (Pack, 2014)

The prevalence of secondary traumatic stress among therapists has been extensively researched to delineate the key variables compounding the impact of traumatic exposure during the course of therapy on the therapist (Stamm, 2005). The individual therapist's degree of identification with the survivor client, the history of the therapist's own victimization and the frequency and duration of exposure to contact with traumatic material in the course of one's work with survivor clients are compounding variables. The motivation for therapists to seek help is another variable in the development in secondary traumatic stress.

For example, the willingness of the therapist to engage in developing a greater awareness of one's process is central to resilience or the ability to 'bounce back' from the secondary trauma encountered. The professional quality of life scale (Stamm, 2005) is one of the self-help tools used to assess the impact of trauma on the therapist. The ProQOL-III (professional equality of life scale) highlights factors impacting a professional helper's quality of life to bring these into conscious awareness so that they can be creatively addressed and actively worked with. (See links to the ProQOL-III in the resources section at the end of this chapter.)

## Vicarious traumatization

The concept of vicarious traumatization refers to the transformation of the professional helper's sense of self, beliefs and world view through their empathetic engagement with traumatic disclosures (McCann and Pearlman, 1990). Put more simply, bearing witness to personal narratives of suffering from survivors puts us at risk of travelling a parallel process of traumatization to our clients. Ironically, the risks of vicarious traumatization are considered to be cumulative and to increase over time (Pearlman and Saakvitne, 1995).

The notion that beliefs and value system combine to influence our thinking as 'cognitive constructs' is at the base of this concept of vicarious traumatization (McCann and Pearlman, 1990). Grounded in the framework of 'constructivist self-development theory', Pearlman and Saakvitne (1995) asked large samples of psychologists to rank lists of statements reflective of the individual's thinking and beliefs about a number of domains of life with a focus on foundational values, cognitions and behaviour indicating changes since commencing work as a sexual abuse therapist in the North American context. This research produced groundbreaking evidence supporting the idea that participants were adversely affected by immersion in traumatic disclosures from their sexually abused clients over time. The effects were discernible in changes in a number of dimensions. These dimensions included relationships, the therapists' sense of self in the world, trust of others (particularly of men due to the statistics on victimization and offending), sense of security and control, world view and social/community engagement (Pearlman and Saakvitne, 1995).

## Compassion fatigue

The professional helper's empathetic responses to disclosures of trauma through the desire to help the other have been termed by Figley and colleagues as 'compassion fatigue': a secondary traumatic stress disorder experienced by trauma professionals. Self-administered questionnaires have been developed to assess the condition that is based in the helper's compassionate response to clients through efforts to assist and help. Compassion fatigue is thought to be akin to a specific form of secondary post-traumatic stress that is routinely experienced by a range of human service workers who have repeated exposure to client trauma. The potential for compassion fatigue is recognized by a range of social service workers, including fire, police emergency personnel and trauma therapists (Figley, 1995). Age, gender and experience of the professional helper have all been discovered to be variables in the development of compassion fatigue, which also is considered to apply to trauma therapists. Being a woman, who is younger or less experienced, providing sexual abuse treatment and length of time doing trauma therapy have all been identified as factors likely to contribute as risk factors to the onset and development of compassion fatigue (Craig and Sprang, 2010; Cunningham, 2003). A history of being traumatized in one's personal biography when this has yet to be explored in personal therapy is thought to be another variable contributing to compassion fatigue. The use of clinical supervision, personal therapy and ongoing professional networks and training, therefore, are identified as factors to ameliorate it (Schauben and Frazer, 1995).

The primary pathway to the onset of compassion fatigue is through the therapist's empathy for the client. The hallmarks of compassion fatigue as a specialized kind of helper second-ary traumatic stress are based in symptoms suggestive of secondary traumatic stress, such as emotional lability and outbursts, anxiety, withdrawal and insomnia (Craig and Sprang, 2010). To assess how engagement with trauma-related work is impacting, the Compassion Fatigue Inventory is useful to periodically complete. This self-administered questionnaire can be found at: http://ncwwi.org/files/Incentives__Work_Conditions/Compassion-Satisfaction-Fatigue-Self-Test.pdf. For useful information and self-administered questionnaires for self-assessment of compassion fatigue, see also Stamm (2005) in the resources at the end of this chapter.

## Transference/countertransference and survivor–therapist issues

Helping professionals' own experiences of trauma have been found to colour their emotional responses in face-to-face dealings with survivor clients. It is common for therapists to enter training with some personal issues yet to resolve, which has been related to the concept of the 'wounded healer' (Sedgwick, 1995). The 'wounded healer' is a term relating to one who tries to help themselves in the course of helping others though not being aware of this moti-vation (Sedgwick, 1995). Sedgwick (1995) asserts that once this awareness is developed then therapists may use their own countertransference as a resource and protective factor in the work.

The consensus of opinion from the research literature is the therapist's responses to what they are hearing daily from their clients in therapy is related to vicarious traumatization through the nexus of the transference/countertransference dyad (Gelso and Hayes, 2007). The classical Freudian view of countertransference is that the therapist's responses to each client stem from the unresolved and unconscious, however, the integrative view that has been evolved is that the therapist response encompasses the responses to the client's trans-ferred and disowned feelings as well as the actual traumatic material (Dalenberg, 2000). This integrative view of countertransference is towards the notion that it is the sum total of the therapist's reactions both now and from projected material from the past that inevi-tably impact (Dalenberg, 2000). This less traditional view of countertransference enables therapists' responses to trauma to be associated more closely to the experience of burnout, vicarious traumatization and the impact of traumatic stress in the present.

Wilson *et al.* (2001) from their research discovered that therapist responses to engage-ment with trauma range on a continuum from those whose tendency is to avoid emotional engagement at one end of the spectrum to those who are overinvolved in the client's trauma at the other. As one can imagine, countertransference responses will be quite different depending on where one is at any one moment on this continuum of therapist countertrans-ference responses. The implications for the development of vicarious traumatization and burnout for those whose engagement forms an over-identification with the client, is likely to more easily be impacted by the traumatic disclosures. Whereabouts a therapist is on this avoidance/over-identification continuum may be influenced by one's experience of trauma-tization, including past trauma, sexual abuse and neglect. A second factor in determining the impact of trauma on the self of the therapist is the openness to explore one's experiences of past trauma in contexts such as personal therapy (Gelso and Hayes, 2007).

## Changes to cognitive patterns

The connecting themes in the use of the terms 'burnout' and 'secondary traumatization' are in relation to the cognitive changes that occur when therapists engage empathetically with their clients who freely disclose their experiences, including traumatic experiences. These signs may or may not be directly attributable to client work, but may be related to triggering issues in the individual therapist's own personal biography, their history of trauma and frequency of exposure to contact with traumatic material. These responses are different from actual experiences of traumatization that therapists might also encounter, as one of the research participants whom I interviewed for my research explained to me.

Sophia, one of the counsellor-participants who works as a psychotherapist, describes some of her indirect experiences of being traumatized. She explains in the following excerpt from an interview, an experience of being vicariously traumatized by client disclosure and her empathetic response (Pack, 2009). Recalling that same incident at interview she remembered the acute nausea and vomiting as a response to hearing a client account:

> Sophia: It was about a little girl that had been raped by her father since the age of four until the age of seven years. And then a multiple rape by thirteen teenagers and she couldn't walk because of it [deep sigh]. And I felt so ill afterwards I actually puked. I mean, just looking at her. If I think about her right now my stomach will hurt and I will have that same feeling – not as intense but just so sad for her, how incredibly hard her life will be.

## Early experiences of trauma

The prevalence of helping professionals entering the fields of mental health and police with early traumatic histories has been analysed in previous studies (Folette *et al.*, 1994; Pope and Feldman-Summers, 1992). A national survey of 500 psychologists in North America found that a third of the participants had some experience of sexual or physical abuse as a child or adolescent (Pope and Feldman-Summers, 1992). This finding was mirrored in the national survey of 558 mental health and law enforcement personnel by Folette *et al.* (1994). This study revealed that 29.8 per cent of the therapists surveyed and 19.6 per cent of the police officers who participated in the research reported some form of childhood trauma. Therefore, therapists who are more open to acknowledging their own issues and responses to clients, including making connections with the present and past experiences, are more likely to seek help for their issues. This awareness is considered to be important to maintaining professional effectiveness as a trauma therapist over time. Seeking a variety of supportive relationships in peer and clinical supervision is vital to ensuring that therapists have an ongoing place to reflect upon the impact of the work on their own selves and lives over the course of a career (Pack, 2009).

Two American psychotherapists who work primarily in private practice in the North American context, Neumann and Gamble (1995: 342), suggest that therapists who are themselves survivors of childhood trauma are likely to identify more closely with their clients, feeling that they are 'thrown into a maelstrom with no lifeline'. Pearlman and Saakvitne (1995) suggest that therapists who are trauma survivors have special needs to attend to and recommend ongoing personal therapy while undertaking therapy with clients as the potential for over-identification with clients leading to a host of complications requires a heightened awareness of self in the practitioner role.

## Compassion satisfaction

Compassion fatigue research has more recently focused attention on the allied term of 'compassion satisfaction' (Stamm, 2005) and 'posttraumatic growth' (Putterman, 2005). These terms expand the scope of compassion fatigue to encompass the idea that, over time, trauma therapists' engagement with trauma inspires a greater appreciation of life in general and reported satisfaction in the work. Specialized trauma training and clinical supervision have been found to ameliorate the more negative impact of trauma therapy on therapists, as they enable therapists to evolve more positive meanings of providing trauma-related psychological intervention (Rich, 1997).

Another counsellor-participant describes how hearing the stories of survivors brings home to her an emancipatory potential that transforms her own life. Hope generated by respect and awe (in a spiritual sense) was evoked for her in witnessing the healing journey of her clients from sexual abuse:

> Jill: It's a balance between the terribleness of it and the awful, awful stories that you hear and the amazement of people, what they've made of their lives. Something quite different and their values. I mean I'm hugely affected by these [stories] but they're really amazing. I'm constantly in awe, really, of some of the stories because, I mean, some I have to say: 'How on earth is this person still alive really?' 'What is holding them?' There's some creative spirit that they keep moving forward.
>
> (Pack, 2009)

## Protective factors promoting post-traumatic growth and resilience

For trauma therapists, the demands of high caseloads, high acuity and client turnover coupled with daily challenging of the conventional medical model of assessment and treatment through a systemic and environmental approach operate to produce a host of potential stressors in the workplace (Pack, 2014). These stressors extend beyond the therapists' clients and their individual experience of traumatization to their interactions with the systems in which they work. In a study of hospital-based therapists, for example, the therapists interviewed for the study were found to balance 'an internal tightrope between empathetic connection with families and emotional separation' in the organizational ethos of 'quick fix' to manage burgeoning caseloads (Badger *et al.*, 2008: 70). 'Preservation methods' were proposed, which suggested that workers make a conscious effort to detach themselves from the patient's experience to self-protect to gain a greater awareness of their own experience to avoid becoming lost within the various pressures (Badger *et al.*, 2008: 70). A regular forum for processing/debriefing and attending to self-care together with finding a work–leisure balance were found to be important to ameliorating the effects of trauma-related work in the hospital context (Badger *et al.*, 2008: 70).

Humour has been found to be a protective factor in moderating vicarious traumatization as it enables helping professionals to cognitively reframe and reinterpret situations and so reduce stress and tension through communication and emotional expression (Moran, 2002: 140–51). However, using humour requires a context in which differing forms of humour are tolerated. As the author comments, 'laughter in the face of tragedy is viewed with suspicion' (Moran, 2002: 140). Maintaining an attitude of 'optimistic perseverance' in the face of difficulties encountered on the job and in relation to client disclosures is similarly recommended (Medeiros and Prochaska, 1988). The development of spirituality and growth of awareness of the intangible humanistic aspects of existence when dealing with trauma is an area of growing interest in developing resilience for helping professionals (e.g. Spiers, 2001). We will address the role of lifestyle, spirituality and belonging in community in Chapters 8 and 9.

Providing opportunities for communicating the experience of the work in clinical supervision is recommended in the range of strategies for enabling therapists to maintain a fresh perspective in the work with trauma survivors (Knight, 2006). The vicarious traumatization and countertransference cycle in the area of worker self-disclosure and boundaries for survivor therapists has illuminated the need to develop specific models of clinical supervision for workers who deal with trauma (Etherington, 2000). These models simultaneously focus on the therapist, the client and supervisees' experience of their work in clinical supervision and the therapists' own personal therapy (Etherington, 2000; Knight, 2006).

## Balancing risk with resilience

Much has been written about how children thrive despite difficult circumstances, yet little has been written about the resilience in adults and specifically those adults working as therapists who engage in trauma. While the concepts of compassion satisfaction and post traumatic growth mentioned earlier do connect with the notion of resilience, there has been a paucity of systematic and empirical evidence of what promotes resilience for therapists as individuals (Pack, 2014). Personality characteristics found associated with the ability to thrive in situations of stress more generally, have been consistently reported as positive adaptations to change, resourcefulness, flexibility and reflectiveness. Engaging proactively in new situations using problem-solving and troubleshooting to find a way forward is reported among the behavioural adaptations promoting psychological hardiness to stress and trauma (Collins, 2007: 257). Beyond simply coping, there is the phenomenon of therapists' immersion in trauma enabling the evolution of values and personal philosophies that are associated with positive feelings and satisfaction linked to the emotional rewards of the work. There are many factors emerging from recent studies on this phenomenon that have been linked to the work on human resilience more generally. Bonnano (2004) found posttraumatic growth in populations facing traumatic loss in situations as diverse as long-term couples facing bereavement to the traumatic losses of family in the 9/11 disaster. Bonnano and colleagues (2011) assert that the normal grieving process together with appropriate support can lead to an expanded capacity to live life well and focus on enhancing satisfaction of life in the longer term. Further findings were that only one-third of all such populations need formal external intervention in the form of counselling to enable a return to everyday life (Bonnano, 2004).

Such optimistic research findings have spurred empirical studies to discover whether there is a similar experience of resilience for those therapists who engage daily in trauma. For example, self-reports by therapists of using evidence-based practices have been associated with post-traumatic growth and resilience in recent studies (Craig and Sprang, 2010). A random sample of 2000 practitioners asked if the self-reported use of evidence-based practices predicted greater compassion satisfaction, and reduced burnout and compassion fatigue. Using the ProQOL-III (Stamm, 2005), nearly half the clinicians surveyed reported high levels of compassion satisfaction (Craig and Sprang, 2010). Practitioners who worked in inpatient settings were found to experience more burnout than did community mental health workers. This survey discovered that the use of evidence-based practice did reduce burnout and compassion fatigue and enhanced compassion satisfaction. The authors surmise that the use of evidence-based practices assists therapists to set appropriate and consistent boundaries with their clients and navigate a pathway through ambiguous and often confusing clinical situations (Craig and Sprang, 2010).

Risk factors predicting burnout included being younger, having a higher percentage of traumatized individuals on one's caseload and not using evidence-based practices. Predictors of compassion satisfaction included the number of years of clinical practice and use of evidence-based practices with clients (Craig and Sprang, 2010). These findings concur with previous research by Cunningham (2003) whose research suggested that maturity and professional experience buffers therapists from the more negative impact of engagement with clients who are making traumatic disclosures. The level of empathetic engagement is another variable that is of interest in the development of vicarious traumatization and compassion fatigue (Figley, 1995; McCann and Pearlman, 1990).

The work environment and the way one is seen by colleagues in the workplace are further variables identified in resilience among trauma therapists. The workload, perceived value of one's work by self and others, and self-concept have been related to therapist resilience and growth (Gibbons *et al.*, 2011). These factors have been found to impact upon positive growth and resilience. Other factors such as role clarity and professional role identity and professional self-esteem are also thought to influence the potential for experiencing post-traumatic growth and compassion satisfaction (Gelso and Hayes, 2007). It is thought that high job satisfaction can lead to positive self-concept and growth for those who engage with traumatized service users though further research is needed to establish this connection (Gibbons *et al.*, 2011).

## Conclusion

There are areas of overlap in the concepts of vicarious traumatization, compassion fatigue and burnout but each has distinguishing differences. The process of vicarious traumatization often involves a process of traumatic countertransference. Countertransference, therefore, is an important process in considering the range of factors that ameliorate or compound the processes of burnout and vicarious traumatization. An awareness of self and the transformation that is occurring in one's personal life is critical to assessing what is occurring. An integrative view of countertransference suggests that most strong emotional responses we have when seeing a client as a therapist constitute a countertransference reaction. Therefore, if we reflect in sufficient depth with a trusted peer or clinical supervisor on what these responses are, connections can be made within the therapist's biography of the present with the past. Within such a view of countertransference being the process leading to or ameliorating vicarious traumatization, the therapist and the client's relationship and inter-subjectivity are acknowledged as the therapeutic relationship is seen as a co-created space.

Coming to terms with one's own traumatic experiences is a theme of the research findings on resilience. Over half of the counsellor-participants I interviewed for my research had experienced traumatic events, including sexual abuse, in their past (Pack, 2009, 2014). This theme is similarly reflected in the literature of helping professionals disclosing traumatic personal histories (Folette *et al.*, 1994; Pope and Feldman-Summers, 1992). They had discovered that their own healing from these experiences was instrumental in guiding their work with traumatized clients. When past traumatic experience was worked through, positive outcomes for clients in therapy with them became possible. In the course of therapy with clients, the counsellor-participants described drawing on a vast pool of intuitive wisdom and knowledge gained in their own personal therapy to guide their work with clients. Their experiential insights, arising from their healing from traumatic experiences, were described as being more important than any of the theories propounded in psychological textbooks by the counsellor-participants. They used this knowledge to engage in social and political action to address the societal myths about abuse and to work actively towards greater social equity (Pack, 2004). In Chapter 2 we turn to learn more about how the counsellor-participants developed personal philosophies and ways of being conducive to remaining fresh for work in the field of trauma therapy over time.

## Resources

### *Self-assessment checklist*

The following checklist (adapted from Rich, 1997) is provided as a personal 'stock take' or audit on how you are dealing with trauma in your work/personal life at any moment in time. Therefore, each time you complete it you have some indication about how trauma and stress may be impacting. Thinking about each statement, highlight any responses you feel strongly resonate with you or if you have noticed a change over time. Discuss your responses to this checklist with a trusted clinical supervisor, your personal therapist, or a colleague or peer who engages in trauma-related work.

Themes in your responses will suggest whether vicarious traumatization is impacting and how this might be affecting your life currently. Jot down any notes, examples or comments about how each statement applies in the spaces provided or use another page if you wish to write down an extended comment or personal reflection. It could be that there are some areas needing further attention within the supervision of your practice. Training on vicarious traumatization may be appropriate or a return to study to learn more about trauma-informed theory. Debriefing from a specific traumatic event encountered in your current work might be needed even when this may have occurred months or years ago. Some of your responses might suggest that a change in work–life balance is highlighted or alternatively a greater variety of client presentation is needed in your current caseload.

1  My formal training prepared me adequately for the work that I do.
2  I went to work in this field to try to right the traumatic wrongs in my own past.
3  I listen to individuals who recount traumatic material about their lives in the course of my work.
4  I believe I experience vicarious traumatization.
5  I feel safe at work.
6  I feel safe when I am at home.
7  I trust other people as much as I ever trusted them since I started doing trauma therapy.
8  I have endured a traumatic experience while doing my present job.
9  If I know a television programme or movie is about trauma, I avoid viewing it.
10  My co-workers seem to understand and support the kind of work I do.
11  I have more frequent nightmares since starting this job.
12  I am a survivor of trauma in my own childhood.
13  I no longer see the world as a meaningful or orderly place since doing this job.
14  I have sought therapy since beginning to work as a trauma therapist.
15  The nature of the work impacts upon my sex life.
16  Since taking this job I have taken a self-defence class.
17  Images of traumatic material intrude into my home time.

18  I enjoy life as much as I ever did before starting this work.
19  I feel confident in my ability to make a difference in my world.
20  I am beginning to see men more negatively since doing this work.
21  I worry more about the safety of my family since I started this work.
22  It has been more difficult to make friends since I commenced this work.
23  Other professionals value the work I do and let me know.
24  I find my work as rewarding as I ever did.
25  I actively believe and practise my spiritual beliefs/religious values in my everyday life.
26  I feel guilty when I hear about what others have endured in the course of my work.
27  I use alcohol and drugs more often since I started this work.
28  The system (police, forensic doctors, courts) as it is works well to help my clients.
29  I use a range of coping strategies (e.g. absorbing interests and hobbies, leisure pursuits, exercise, listening to music and being in nature, etc).
30  I tend to avoid or delay working on my more traumatic cases.
31  I am less compassionate than I was before taking this job.
32  I find it difficult not to over-identify with the victim/survivor of traumatic events.
33  I tend to avoid going out at night by myself.
34  I have been involved in court/legal proceedings in the course of doing my job.
35  I find it difficult not to feel angry towards perpetrators.
36  I am more anxious since starting this work.
37  I feel like I have failed if any of my clients are harmed.
38  Since doing this work I feel somewhat removed from my circle of friends and family.
39  I have experienced flashbacks/intrusive memories of my client's traumas.
40  I feel more isolated/alone in doing the work I do.
41  I find I feel more depressed/sad since engaging with this work.
42  I am more cautious in trusting new people I meet in my personal life.
43  I believe the work I do will make a difference in people's lives.
44  My professional association/union are places I feel I can go to for support and information about my rights and responsibilities in my job.
45  People say about my work: 'how can you listen to such terrible things day after day' or 'I couldn't do that'.
46  I see therapy as being as effective as I used to.
47  I often feel isolated and different because of the work I do.
48  I feel frustrated when faced with the apparent inactivity of other institutions who are involved with my clients.
49  I have a range of resources to manage the strains of my job.
50  Empowering trauma survivors empowers me.

## *Weblinks*

www.isst-d.org  International Society for the Study of Trauma and Dissociation (ISST)

An international not-for-profit organization aiming to develop and promote empirically sound resources and education on complex trauma and dissociation. The ISST offers professional development and training programmes, webinars, professional conferences and the *Journal of Trauma and Dissociation*. Its mission is to advance knowledge and understanding in society of the prevalence and consequences of chronic trauma and dissociation from the professional's perspective.

Options to follow on Facebook and Twitter

www.anzatsa.org Australian and New Zealand Association for the Treatment of Sexual Abuse (ANZATSA)

An Australasian professional association committed to protecting the community through the promotion of professional standards, practices and education in sexual abuse prevention, assessment, intervention and research. ANZATSA runs annual conferences and the *Journal of the Sociological Association of Aotearoa (NZ)*, and offers ongoing professional development and training. Members promote abuse prevention, education in child protection, child education, community education and professional education. Members work within the disciplines of psychology, psychiatry and social work.

# References

American Psychiatric Association. (2013). *Diagnostic and statistical manual of mental disorders* (5th edn). Washington, DC: Author.

Badger, K., Royse, D. and Craig, C. (2008). Hospital social workers and indirect trauma exposure: An exploratory study of contributing factors. *Health and Social Work, 33* (1), 63–71. doi: 10.1093/hsw/33.1.63.

Bonnano, G. A. (2004). Loss, trauma, and human resilience: Have we underestimated the human capacity to thrive after extremely aversive events? *American Psychologist, 59* (1), 20–8. doi: 10.1037/0003-066x.59.1.20

Bonnano, G. A., Westphal, M. and Mancini, A. D. (2011). Resilience to loss and potential trauma. *Annual Review of Clinical Psychology, 7* (1), 511–35. doi: 10.1146/annurev-clinpsy-032210-104526

Collins, S. (2007). Social workers' resilience, positive emotions and optimism. *Practice: Social Work in Action, 19* (4), 255–69. doi: 10.1080/09503150701728186

Craig, C. D. and Sprang, G. (2010). Compassion satisfaction, compassion fatigue, and burnout in a national sample of trauma treatment therapists. *Anxiety, Stress and Coping, 23* (3), 319–39. doi: 10.1080/10615800903085818

Cunningham, M. (2003). Impact of trauma work on social work clinicians: Empirical findings. *Social Work, 48* (4), 451–9. doi: 10.1093/sw/48.4.451

Dalenberg, C. (2000). *Countertransference and the treatment of trauma.* La Jolla, CA: American Psychological Association.

Etherington, K. (2000). Supervising counsellors who work with survivors of childhood sexual abuse. *Counselling Psychology Quarterly, 13* (4), 377–89. doi: 10.1080/713658497

Figley, C. R. (1995). *Compassion fatigue.* New York: Brunner/Mazel.

Folette, V. M., Polusny, M. M. and Milbeck, K. (1994). Mental health and law enforcement professionals: Trauma history, psychological symptions and the impact of providing services to child sexual abuse survivors. *Professional Psychology Research and Practice, 25* (3), 275–82. doi: 10.1037/0735-7028.25.3.275

Fulcher, L. C. (1988). *The worker, the work team and the organisational task: Corporate re-structuring and the social services in New Zealand.* Wellington: Victoria University Press.

Gelso, C. J. and Hayes, J. (2007). *Countertransference and the therapist's inner experience: Perils and possibilities.* Mahwah, NJ: Lawrence Erlbaum.

Gibbons, S., Murphy, D. and Joseph, S. (2011). Countertransference and positive growth in social workers. *Journal of Social Work Practice, 25* (1), 17–30. doi: 10.1080/02650530903579246

Grauerholz, L. (2000). An ecological approach to understanding sexual re-victimisation: Linking personal, interpersonal and sociocultural factors and processes. *Child Maltreatment, 5* (2), 5–17.

Grosch, W. N. and Olsen, D. C. (1994). *When helping starts to hurt: A new look at burnout among psychotherapists.* New York: Norton.

Harms, L. (2015). *Understanding trauma and resilience.* London: Palgrave Macmillan.

Herman, J. (1992). *Trauma and recovery: The aftermath of violence – From domestic abuse to political terror*. New York: Basic Books.

Herman, J. (2010). *Trauma and recovery: The aftermath of violence – From domestic abuse to political terror* (2nd edn, reprint). London: Pandora.

Knight, C. (2006). Working with survivors of childhood trauma. *The Clinical Supervisor*, *23* (2), 81–105. doi: 10.1300/j001v23n02_06

Leiter, M. P. and Maslach, C. (1988). The impact of interpersonal environment on burnout and organisational commitment. *Journal of Organisational Behaviour*, *9* (4), 297–308. doi: 10.1002/job.4030090402

McCann, I. L. and Pearlman, L. A. (1990). Vicarious traumatisation: A framework for understanding the psychological effects of working with victims. *Journal of Traumatic Stress*, *3* (1), 131–49. doi: 10.1002/jts.2490030110

Medeiros, M. E. and Prochaska, J. O. (1988). Coping strategies that psychotherapists use in working with stressful clients. *Professional Psychology: Research and Practice*, *19*, 112–14. doi: 10.1037//0735-7028.19.1.112

Moran, C. C. (2002). Humor as a moderator of compassion fatigue. In C. R. Figley (Ed.), *Treating compassion fatigue* (pp. 139–54). New York: Brunner-Routledge.

Neumann, D. A. and Gamble, S. J. (1995). Issues in the professional development of psychotherapists: Countertransference and vicarious traumatisation in the new therapist. *Psychotherapy*, *32* (2), 341–7. doi: 10.1037/0033-3204.32.2.341

Pack, M. J. (2004). Sexual abuse counsellors' responses to stress and trauma: A social work perspective. *New Zealand Journal of Counselling*, *25* (2), 1–17. Retrieved from www.nzac.org.nz/new_zealand_journal_of_counselling.cfm (accessed 16 March 2016)

Pack, M. J. (2009). The body as a site of knowing: Sexual abuse therapists' experiences of stress and trauma. *Women's Study Journal*, *23* (2), 46–56. Retrieved from www.wsanz.org.nz (accessed 16 March 2016)

Pack, M. (2014). Vicarious resilience: A multilayered model of stress and trauma. *Affilia: Journal of Women and Social Work*, *29* (1), 18–29. doi: 10.1177/0886109913510088

Pearlman, L. A. and Saakvitne, K. W. (1995). *Trauma and the therapist: Countertransference and vicarious traumatisation in psychotherapy with incest survivors*. New York: Norton.

Pope, K. S. and Feldman-Summers, S. (1992). National survey of psychologists' sexual and physical abuse history and their evaluation of training and competence in these areas. *Professional Psychology: Research and Practice*, *23* (5), 353–61. doi: 10.1037//0735-7028.23.5.353

Putterman, I. (2005). The relationship between posttraumatic growth and professional quality of life (compassion fatigue/secondary trauma, compassion satisfaction and burnout) among social workers in Texas (Unpublished doctoral dissertation). Houston, TX: University of Houston.

Rich, K. D. (1997). Vicarious traumatisation: A preliminary study. In S. B. Edmunds (Ed.), *Impact: Working with sexual abusers* (pp. 75–88). Brandon, Vermont: Safer Society Press.

Schauben, L. J. and Frazer, P. A. (1995). Vicarious trauma: The effects on female counsellors of working with sexual violence survivors. *Psychology of Women Quarterly*, *19* (1), 49–64. doi: 10.1111/j.1471-6402.1995.tb00278.x

Sedgwick, D. (1995). *The wounded healer: Countertransference from a Jungian perspective*. London: Routledge.

Spiers, T. (Ed.). (2001). *Trauma: A practitioner's guide to counselling*. New York: Brunner-Routledge.

Stamm, B. H. (2005). *The ProQOL manual: Professional quality of life scale – Compassion satisfaction, burnout and compassion fatigue/secondary trauma scales*. Retrieved from www.compassionfatigue.org/pages/ProQOLManualOct05.pdf (accessed 28 February 2016).

van Heugten, K. (2011). *Social work under pressure: How to overcome stress, fatigue and burnout in the workplace*. London: Jessica Kingsley.

Wall, L. and Quadara, A. (2014). Acknowledging the complexity in the impacts of sexual victimisation trauma. *Australian Centre for the Study of Sexual Assault Newsletter*, *16*. Retrieved from www3.aifs.gov.au/acssa/pubs/issue/i16/ (accessed 28 February 2016).

Wilson, J. P., Friedman, M. J. and Lindy, J. D. (Eds). (2001). *Treating psychological trauma and PTSD*. New York: Guilford Press.

# Chapter 2 **Discovering what builds resilience in trauma therapists**

## Findings from earlier research and reflections on practice

### Introduction

I find pathologising discourse pretty unhelpful to my clients. And most of the psychological papers or theories are purely psychological discourse. So anything that is prescriptive or diagnostic around me or may pathologise me or other psychologists or therapists I'd avoid just as much as I would for my clients. That's why I think this article [McCann and Pearlman, 1990] is quite interesting. It sits quite comfortably alongside that book I mentioned [White, 1997]. Which is about the opposite of traumatising therapists. It is about how therapists that are exposed to a lot of trauma and difficulties actually overcome them.

In some ways from a personal and professional viewpoint we need to learn from those therapists who have been exposed to a lot of this kind of work how they sustain themselves and how they manage to have a full life and help people in ways that are helpful and are also helpful to themselves.

*David, one of the counsellor-participants explains his personal philosophy incorporating an understanding of the quality of relationship between himself and his clients when dealing with traumatic disclosures*

This chapter reports the findings of a qualitative research study that explores trauma therapists' theories for practice and how they say they develop and use an array of theoretical approaches to support their well-being and clinical effectiveness over time (Pack, 2004, 2009a, 2010b, 2014). This research contextualizes the concepts of vicarious traumatization and resilience. Half the sample of 22 government-contracted Accident Compensation Corporation (ACC)-registered therapists were trained in other professions than counselling and psychotherapy prior to entering the field. The findings suggest that trauma therapists who engage with traumatic disclosures from their clients actively evolve strategies and resources that act to buffer the more negative effects of the work with sexual abuse survivors, which is a means of ameliorating vicarious traumatization.

The negative orientation of the vicarious traumatization framework has recently been challenged as trauma therapists over time have been discovered to evolve ways of being that are protective of their personal well-being and professional effectiveness (Gelso and Hayes,

2007; Steed and Downing, 1998). In this chapter, I explore the historical background and context to the theoretical eclecticism described by the participants interviewed for research I undertook as my doctorate in social work. The findings suggest that the practitioners' reference to theory is both a resource and protective factor that is drawn upon to support the day-to-day work of sexual abuse therapy. This chapter therefore draws from a larger study of counsellor stress and trauma that triangulated the responses of the counsellor-participants with the perceptions of their nominated family, friends and colleagues (Pack, 2004, 2009a, 2010a, 2010b) The findings of this research regarding the therapists' significant others will be discussed in Chapter 4.

While there was little theory specific to trauma work in the early 1980s when the research participants were first practising, they developed a framework for their practice based in a combination of early training, practice and personal experiences. These developed insights and reference to diverse strands of theory together constitute a framework for practice that assists the counsellors' in their understanding of their clients, the dynamics of the therapeutic relationship, organisational constraints on funding that surround their work and their own self care. The theoretical frameworks that the participants preferred to use derive from social justice principles, feminist, narrative theories and the 'New Trauma Therapy' (Coffey 1998). An example from my own practice concludes the chapter. Recommendations for clinician self-care in dealing with traumatic disclosures with reference to a range of theoretical approaches are suggested from an extended reflection of practice with trauma survivors.

## The context of trauma therapy in New Zealand

Citizens in New Zealand have the availability of a 24-hour, 7-days-a-week, no-fault comprehensive personal injury insurance cover through the Accident Compensation Corporation of New Zealand (ACC). Anyone who has experienced sexual abuse or assault in New Zealand can lodge a claim for mental injury, known as a 'sensitive claim' (ACC, 2015).

ACC-funded therapy services are delivered by a range of providers based around New Zealand, many of whom are private practitioners of various disciplines (counsellors, psychologists, psychotherapists and social workers) who are registered by the ACC as providers of treatment for trauma survivors.

The public can search through the Register of Approved Counsellors through an external web-link to find a therapist based on location, field of expertise, speciality, culture, gender and language. The search results will show also the details of organizations with therapists that meet the ACC's registration criteria. These criteria for registration of the professionals who are listed in the register involve specialized training in trauma assessment and therapy.

The recent media reports of changes to processes for ACC funding for sexual abuse has highlighted the important role publicly funded therapy has for the survivors of violence to regain their quality of life (Hayward, 2009; Kay, 2009). These reports in the media indicate the importance the issue of trauma and trauma recovery has in the New Zealand public's consciousness.

## Background: the context of therapy for sexual abuse survivors in Aotearoa

In New Zealand, sexual abuse therapy is publicly funded as survivors of sexual abuse trauma are covered under the ACC which provides funded psychotherapy to claimants with an accepted sensitive claim. Once a sensitive claim is accepted, claimants are able to obtain counselling as one of the main methods of recovery from trauma. An increasing range of counselling professionals including clinical psychologists, psychotherapists and social workers have chosen to register to provide this specialized service.

The public funding of therapy for sexual abuse survivors represented to the counsellor-participants a double-edged sword. Reporting requirements of the ACC were considered by the research participants interviewed to hold the potential for episodic disruptions in the therapeutic relationship they held with their clients which they constructed as a collaborative endeavour by witnessing their clients' narratives. These reporting requirements were found to be the major challenge in working within the field from the counsellor-participants' perspectives as it meant that they were required to move out of a relational mode of being with the client to reporting the details of their clients' abuse and biography to determine eligibility for ongoing funding of therapy. Sometimes this meant that they needed to delineate the part of the abuse that was covered by the sensitive claim, so that a specific event could be actively worked with to secure eligibility for ongoing public funding.

The requirement for trauma therapists to determine 'mental injury' to establish the ongoing need for funding was seen as pathologizing the client. Psychotherapists have criticized in the media the ACC's requirement of periodic referral to a psychiatrist to establish mental illness arising from the original event for which the claim has been accepted to secure ongoing funding for treatment (Hayward, 2009). This new 'clinical pathway process' had widespread ramifications to how trauma therapists in New Zealand were able to assist trauma survivors. This change is reflected in the reduction in number of accepted sensitive claims for mental injury resulting from assault. This figure has declined in recent years from 3,991 accepted claims to receive ongoing treatment in 2007, to only 49 sensitive claims accepted for treatment expenses in 2012 (Shuttleworth, 2012). The changes in assessment procedures were held responsible for this dramatic drop in accepted claims providing ongoing funded therapy for sensitive claimants (Shuttleworth, 2012).

The difference in philosophy between the statutory funding requirements and the way practitioners who contract to provide this service say that they work in practice with their clients is also highlighted by these debates. The ACC requirement in which mental injury needs to be established medically at more frequent junctures during the therapy, often involving psychiatric and medical assessment and re-assessment, has been questioned on ethical grounds by the registered counsellors as a group (Hayward, 2009; Kay, 2009). These additional reporting and assessment requirements have been described as 'unethical' due to the restrictions funding conditions impose on the therapist and therapeutic relationship with clients (Hayward, 2009; Kay, 2009).

Recent changes made to the sensitive claims process in response to these concerns now mean that survivors are offered a number of individual sessions in which to determine eligibility if claim cover is in fact needed. Therapists have the option to suggest to the client that they are referred to a social worker or cultural provider approved by the ACC as an alternative option initially to source ongoing help that may not be therapy. On paper at least, this process appears to offer a more flexible approach to dealing with trauma survivors' differing needs. The operational guidelines introduced in 2015 by the ACC are designed to implement the new Integrated Services for Sensitive Claims (ISSC) contract. This service provides some flexibility in whether claimants are seen with the intention of lodging a sensitive claim or whether other kinds of short-term support and discharge or referral for other services are required once the client is seen and assessed. For suppliers of service, this means more discretion can be exercised by the therapist over what kind of services are deemed appropriate for each individual client. The new process also requires individual therapists to 'tender' for service as an ACC supplier of service, and set up as a sole trader through a third-party manager (ACC, 2015).

The formal evaluation of how the contract is working in its operation has yet to be undertaken, yet anecdotally some of the counsellor-participants have made a decision to withdraw from providing therapeutic services after more than 20 years as a registered trauma specialist therapist with the ACC due to needing to set up as a 'sole trader' managed by a third-party manager. For some of the counsellor-participants this requirement after so many changes in policy relating to their work as a therapist was considered 'a step too far' (Beth, counsellor-participant, personal communication, October 2015).

In research I conducted between 1998 and 2002 with ACC-registered therapists, a theme in the in-depth, one-to-one interviews was the lack of recognition of the importance of relationship in the way the funding arrangements worked in practice (Pack, 2004, 2009a). For the therapists interviewed about vicarious traumatization, they described the part of their job they found the most 'traumatizing' as managing the statutory reporting and assessment requirements alongside the need to maintain the therapeutic relationship. Under the new ISSC guidelines and processes, the time frame for assessment is more flexible and there is scope for discharging and referring on to other registered therapists, social workers and cultural support workers depending on what the client needs at any one moment in time. Hopefully this will provide some relief to the ethical dilemma of seeing a client whose abuse did not fit the criteria for 'cover' under a sensitive claim as Sally, one of the counsellor-participants, explains:

> Sally: I have had a case just recently, a new client, who in terms of abuse, if you look at it, on a scale of abuse, her abuse may be about a three out of ten, but for her, the effects of the abuse on her life have been ten out of ten. It was hard, in fact, when we were filling out the form as I was thinking: 'Hey, they [ACC] might not pay out on this one, because it's not a biggie in the wider scheme of things'. But in terms of the trauma in the person's life, that's had a life-changing impact. It's not what happened necessarily, it's the effect of what has happened over time.

In light of how the organizational and policy frameworks impacted on the counsellor-participants in the ACC contracting system, I developed a model of vicarious traumatization that included the organizational or structural component, to explain this experience described by the therapists I interviewed. I found that through reference to theory and practice wisdom, the participants also found ways of working creatively within the organizational and funding constraints, however. This chapter, therefore, focuses on the theoretical frameworks that the participants in the study said that they drew upon that acted as a protective factor promoting their resilience in their practice with sexual abuse and trauma survivors.

## Key definitions

As we saw from Chapter 1, vicarious traumatization is a process that occurs when a worker's sense of self and world view is negatively transformed through empathetic engagement with traumatic disclosures from clients (Pearlman and Saakvitne, 1995). The effects are considered to be cumulative, permanent and irreversible if unattended (Pearlman and Saakvitne, 1995). The focus of my research into vicarious traumatization was to discover how trauma therapists working for the ACC navigated the various perils and pitfalls of the work and the organizational context in which they operated to evolve ways of being that maintained their professional effectiveness over the length of their careers. I chose very experienced therapists to interview strategically; most had accrued practice insights over 20–30 years of practice. I was interested to know how the counsellor-participants managed to keep a fresh perspective upon their practice with trauma survivors despite the negative cautioning of the vicarious traumatization literature.

## Factors promoting therapist resilience

Against this organizational backdrop, recent studies have discovered that the presence of protective factors operate to mitigate the negative impact of the work with trauma on the practitioner (Gelso and Hayes, 2007). These factors include the counsellor's ability to actively access and use social supports, deal with organizational stressors present in their workplaces and moderate their own empathy to regulate emotional responsiveness (Badger *et al.*, 2008). Strategies including the use of collegial and personal support, clinical supervision and personal therapy have all been discussed in relation to what promotes worker resilience in the field of trauma recovery from a social work perspective (Badger *et al.*, 2008; Pack, 2004). Knowledge of theoretical approaches facilitates awareness, understanding and integration of the distressing countertransference responses that are evoked in the work with trauma survivors, and provides a further means of making meaning from experience for clinicians (Gelso and Hayes, 2007). Personal insight, conceptualizing skills, empathy, self-integration and anxiety management have been found to be relevant to the well-being of the practitioner who engages with sexual abuse and trauma disclosures (Gelso and Hayes, 2007: 102). Such factors promote therapist resilience (Gelso and Hayes, 2007) which enables the practitioner to 'bounce back' from the usual challenges of trauma-related helping. Therefore, the process by which these conceptualizing skills with reference to theory are evoked in the work with sexual abuse survivors was one of the aims chosen for the research into sexual abuse therapists' experiences of the work (Pack, 2009a).

## Aims of the study

My aim as a researcher with a therapy and social work background was to elicit 'thick description' (Geertz, 1975) on the topic of vicarious traumatization that appeared to be missing in the tradition of research on vicarious traumatization, which originally was developed from survey research by clinical psychologists (McCann and Pearlman, 1990; Pearlman and Saakvitne, 1995). Therefore, I aimed to explore sexual abuse counsellors' views of the vicarious traumatization literature in the New Zealand context by researching the counsellors' viewpoints and practice narratives in response to the original vicarious traumatization framework (Pearlman and Saakvitne, 1995). I also hoped to learn what kept the counsellors going through the rigours of trauma involvement on the job.

## Methodological approach

A qualitative, participative design was chosen to research the question of whether vicarious traumatization was an issue from the individual counsellor's experience of the work. Second, the intention was to discover how the nature of the work with traumatic disclosures had impacted on the family members of the counselors (Pack, 2004, 2009a). Due to the sensitive nature of the topic and the need to elicit in-depth discussion from a narrative perspective, a semi-structured topic guide was developed in liaison with a focus group of currently practising ACC psychotherapists to pretest the relevance of the methodological approach and methods chosen. Second, at the data analysis stage, early themes were presented to the group for discussion and feedback in a way suggested in feminist and participative research methodologies (Reason, 1988; Reinharz, 1992).

## The counsellor-participants

The participants in this research (hereafter referred to as the counsellor-participants) were selected using a systematic sample from the ACC's Register of Approved Counsellors. Therefore, a representative sample of a range of professional groupings within the register (social workers, psychotherapists, counsellors and psychologists) were sought by selecting a range of individuals from several different professional associations. It was discovered once the fieldwork commenced that half the sample held other roles later moving through further training to more specialized trauma psychotherapy and counselling roles (Pack, 2009a, 2010a, 2010b). This career trajectory and background is indicative of many professionals who register to provide ACC sexual abuse therapy in New Zealand and internationally (Pack, 2009a). For example, a generic family therapist in the sample for the research moved into trauma therapy with individuals due to the caseload she developed to align with her therapeutic interests and ongoing training in trauma-informed models of recovery.

## Methods

Twenty-two counsellor-participants were interviewed individually in total, using qualitative research design and methods. Ethical approval from Victoria University of Wellington, New Zealand, was obtained before the project commenced. The data from in-depth interviews was transcribed and analysed thematically, guided by a focus group who acted as consultants throughout the project to verify and analyse emerging themes.

## Data analysis

Similarities and differences within the counsellor narratives were analysed using thematic analysis and 'pattern-matching' (Yin, 1985) in which each interview transcript was analysed for internal consistency and themes. These themes were identified as recurring patterns within the transcripts and then discussed with the focus group to add a further layer of verification. The counsellor-participants chose their own pseudonyms to represent their individual contributions, as previously discussed in the preface to this book.

The relevance of the original vicarious traumatization framework (McCann and Pearlman, 1990) was used to analyse the themes across the counsellor-participants as a group alongside the notion of protective factors leading to therapist resilience, drawn from the risk and resilience literature among trauma therapists (Steed and Downing, 1998).

Thematic analysis to determine patterns in the data, therefore, guided the interpretation of findings together with reference to a focus group (Reason, 1988). To analyse the emerging findings and to avoid the researcher's frame of reference being the only means of verification, a focus group of five currently practising sexual abuse counsellors were involved throughout the project by the organization of monthly meetings. Early themes were discussed for relevancy, and the group's comments were incorporated in the data analysis over the duration of the study in a way that is recommended in participative research approaches (Reason, 1988).

## Findings: a 'baptism by fire'

The current research participants, who were trailblazers in working with those sexually abused in the New Zealand context, referred to the experimental nature of their early work. A consultant to the present study, Ellen, became aware of the prevalence of sexual abuse through her involvement as a media personality in talkback radio and television programmes where viewers wrote and talked to her on air. Later Ellen trained in psychology and became a psychotherapist. This narrative of Ellen's personal journey illustrates the eclecticism of roles and approaches that were evoked by the historical times in which she was working and the dynamic tension between her early training and later on-the-job experiences. For Ellen and the other counsellor-participants, these transformations in outlook and changing times necessitate a reformulation of who one is, what one does and how one engages with clients:

> Ellen: One important lesson that I learned out of this was that one could invite a person whom I was corresponding with, to write in as much detail as they felt safe to or able to do. To either write in detail or to draw what the trauma was or what the pictures were that stayed in their mind. Flashbacks really. And by correspondence we were actually able to work through those. I find it quite extraordinary now looking back on that because I didn't even know that post-traumatic stress disorder existed. I certainly didn't know what the name would be but we were actually working with it then. Now by 1986 I was probably dealing with hundreds of letters, many of them about sexual abuse, incest and from guys in prison who were able to talk about their own abuse but not prepared to talk about it to the authorities, so we have quite a lot of experience then in talking to perpetrators by letter.

The lack of published work and theory to underpin the early efforts of trauma therapists was a theme for the counsellor-participants interviewed. *The Courage to Heal* (Bass and Davis, 1988 and Davis and Bass, 1992), a self-help manual for sexual abuse survivors, was referred to to guide the work. This lack of a coherent theory about trauma and the aftermath set Ellen and the other counsellor-participants in a search for theories and further training that could support their practice.

> Ellen: Even later I became a co-host and dealt with sexual abuse, incest and so on, on air. The issues were widespread; they crossed socio-economic barriers. There was just a very wide exposure to abuse issues throughout the country. However, by 1991, now trained as a psychotherapist, I decided that I wanted to work more in-depth with abused and traumatised clients. And I knew that I was going to be looking at long-term work. And this still continues. In that time I had worked with clients who have been ritually abused as children and DID [dissociative identity disorder] clients and it's been, through working with them, I think, that most of my internal changing would have taken place.

## Theoretical underpinnings to practice

The 'new trauma therapy' (NTT) as proposed by Coffey (1998) and epitomized in the writings of Herman (1992), Briere (1996), Courtois (1997) and Dalenberg (2000), among others, represents the eclecticism that the counsellor-participants discussed as being central to their work with sexual abuse survivors. Theories encompassed by new trauma therapy were discussed as guiding their own healing from traumatic events and recovery from vicarious traumatization. The new trauma therapy is derived from a range of theories and sources. It re-conceptualizes the therapeutic relationship in ways that assist the healing processes of survivors of trauma. It ameliorates the therapists' own experiences of trauma, both their own and vicariously experienced. As Coffey (1998) suggests, a writer who has researched trauma therapists and their work with survivors, the new trauma therapy is a synthesis of Freud and newer theorists. Coffey (1998: 163) refers to the research of trauma theorists Kluft and Gartrell to suggest the potential pitfalls of abandoning established psychotherapeutic practice and approaches when dealing with traumatized clients. Coffey (1998: 163) concludes after interviewing sexual abuse survivors and trauma theorists that 'therapists who toss aside all psychotherapeutic tradition may also unwittingly and perilously toss aside its protections, forcing themselves to blaze unnecessarily chancy paths through precarious jungles'.

The research participants often disliked the need to categorize clients using systems of classification such as the DSM IV-TR, preferring to use approaches drawn from the new trauma therapy in their work with traumatized clients. They viewed these approaches as complementing the traditional psychodynamic models with ideas closer to their own theories and ways of thinking. Herman (1992) and other theorists within the new trauma therapy referred to the historical and social contexts in which people experience trauma. This attention to context and the wider social systems was missing in more individual-focused, medically orientated approaches. This refocusing of attention onto context was itself a product of the historical times in which Herman and the new trauma therapists were witnesses to a culture of disbelief about abuse. Therapy as a political act challenging the disbelief about the prevalence of abuse that exists in society has provided important framing to the disclosures from survivors (Herman, 1992).

In a similar way, the counsellor-participants described responding to the disbelief they encountered within the wider community about the prevalence of sexual abuse in the New Zealand context. They conceptualized their roles as therapists as enabling survivors to regain their voice and their narratives. Within such reclaiming, there is a potential for returning to principles of social justice in approaching sexual abuse and recovery.

Jill, one of the counsellor-participants in the research, for example, expressed reservations about her early training to be a psychotherapist. She found her personal experiences in various experiential, psychodynamic therapy contexts did not fit with her wider analysis of class, gender and oppression. Later, she trained as a social worker and, in being introduced to the writings of Freire (1970), found an alternative model that better fitted with her personal philosophy, as a 'working class' woman. She elaborated her ideas into the concept of therapy as liberation from social/personal oppression. She recalled coming across such theories as 'a homecoming' after years of training in various psychoanalytic/psychodynamic approaches:

> Jill: When I went to do social work training, that was a real homecoming for me and just really reading Freire was the thing, and after that I always felt that I had this touchstone in a way. Because there wasn't really even any feminist counselling material out at that time, that wasn't quite psychodynamic. But I like that idea of Freire's, about being in solidarity with people, as they changed their perception of themselves, as they began to appreciate themselves in this way, and so I always just used that and I still revert to that. And I noticed in a book that's just been published by Freire's wife, after his death, about his thinking on getting on with the oppressed, which was the first book I read, and the first one he wrote, where he was saying that, in fact, that was 'therapy'. What he was talking about was not just liberation theory, it was therapy. And I began to think about therapy as liberation and that was what we were doing really, and that a person needed to be liberated socially in terms of their personal safety but also that your mind has to be liberated as well. And so that's how I've always thought about what I do and still think about it in this way.

Throughout their training, Mary and Beth, another two of the counsellor-participants in the research, described integrating structural and individual perspectives in their work. Both focus on their experiences as women and their experiences in personal therapy as informing how they work with their clients. Being a survivor of abuse or not may not be the central issue here. As Mary suggests, women are all, in a sense, survivors of dominance by patriarchal institutions and relationships. Both Beth and Mary find the 'expert' role as ill fitting their respective approaches with clients with whom they prefer to be in 'partnership' (Beth) or 'in solidarity' (Jill). Their respective visions of the world revolve around working with the wider systems that influence people's lives. These ideas encompass notions of difference and diversity. Sexual abuse is viewed as being one example of the many sources of oppression in society. The role of power in social relationships, including the therapeutic relationship, becomes the primary focus of attention. Such an analysis is not only useful as a tool for personal transformation. It is also useful as the basis for a critical appraisal of one's own practice and the broader context in which therapy takes place.

> Mary: What I am enjoying now about where some of the narrative writers and therapists have got to is the both/and rather than going into dualisms. That the importance of acknowledging (and I need to define problems clearly as well as acknowledging pain) and then offering hope as well. And that comes back full circle with clients into therapy which is really hearing and letting the client know that you are really hearing. I was quite influenced by a statement that I don't know who made it but I first heard it from another therapist. It was something like: the core of counselling is something about not moving somebody on but encouraging the person to be where they are when they themselves are able to be there.

## Discussion

The eclectic and holistic nature of theoretical approaches they espoused enabled the counsellor-participants to keep pace with the transformations they were experiencing in themselves and in relation to their work. Their critical appraisals of earlier training, experiences and personal and professional growth necessitated revisions to their initial conceptualization of the therapeutic relationship. The new trauma therapy conceptualized the therapeutic relationship in ways that were more compatible with these revisions as the concept of 'witnessing' (Herman, 1992) enabled them to adopt a narrative and social justice paradigm in their work alongside other psychodynamically orientated theories. This sense of integrating a diverse range of theories in their practice with sexual abuse survivors was described as a resource in the participants' work enabling them to remain feeling connected to their value base for practice, which is an ameliorating factor in vicarious traumatization (Pack, 2004).

## Implications for therapist well-being

The changes to current ACC sensitive claims protocols focus on the assessment/review and evaluation processes to establish the need for treatment on the basis of mental injury. Counsellor-participants in this study found these processes before the recent proposed changes to be the most challenging part of the role. Being in an uninterrupted relationship with their clients enabled the counsellor-participants to stay connected with their diverse sources of theory, which include an awareness of vicarious traumatization and a political analysis of why abuse occurs in society. On the basis of this awareness, the counsellor-participants had developed and internalized knowledge of how to manage their own trauma and stress effectively, which if unaddressed can accumulate and result in vicarious traumatization over time. The findings suggest that there needs to be realignment of the philosophies of the organizations involved in sexual abuse work towards an approach consistent with the practice of trauma therapists, that is, what trauma therapists actually do in practice with their clients. Based in this research, a synthesis of narrative, anti-oppressive and strengths-based frameworks offers a possible meeting place for organizations and workers to engage in a dialogue on these issues about the assessment and evaluation processes needed to apply for the continued funding of therapy. How this would work through a third-party business manager working with the counsellor-participants in the 2015 changes to the ACC sensitive claim process, is another issue for consideration.

At a time when counselling professionals are under increasing pressure and scrutiny to be effective in producing measurable outcomes, the context in which sexual abuse counselling occurs is defined by its unpredictability. ACC counselling largely defies managerial attempts at control and integration, despite vigorous attempts to the contrary. Paradoxically, larger numbers of survivors are presenting to helping services throughout New Zealand than previously. Services to sexual abuse survivors in the climate of budgetary control and tightening of the public purse strings are increasingly producing diverse and fragmented services that remain largely uncoordinated. In this climate, it becomes difficult for professions such as trauma counsellors and psychotherapists to enact their professions' values or goals. As Fook *et al.* (2000) found in their five-year longitudinal study of social workers, as representatives of the 'caring professions' founded on principles of social justice, it becomes increasingly problematic in the managerial climate of statutory organizations for social workers to begin to know how to begin to practise to embody these principles.

## Conclusion

Trauma therapists are aware that in turning a blind eye to the stories of oppression they hear daily, they risk avoiding the issues of their own vulnerability and the possibility of travelling the same path as survivors to becoming vicariously traumatized. In this sense, therapy is a highly personal and politicized activity that aims to redress the grievances of those whose trust has been deeply betrayed. To locate these abuses as residing in the individual, is a re-enactment of the blaming/denial dynamics of the original abuse. For some therapists uncovering the collective injustices that exist is an unexpected outcome of their witnessing of individual narratives of oppression. Conceptualized this way, the need for emancipatory modes of practice unfolds with the telling and retelling of the individual narrative and the therapists' awareness of the connecting themes within these narratives.

The expectation of practice from an organizational perspective is one based in scientific knowledge that draws cause-and-effect relationships. The presenting problems or issues seem to automatically lead to diagnosis or formulation which then assumes 'treatment' and, ultimately, 'cure'. Such a model of causality fits uneasily when dealing with survivors of trauma from the perspective of the counsellor-participants. This view distances the worker into a role of diagnostic expert. Organizational discourses that are authored within 'residual' or 'maintenance' approaches (Adams *et al.*, 2009: 209–14) need to acknowledge and facilitate the ways in which counsellors and clients relate.

For the therapists who engage with clients recovering from the aftermath of trauma, there is an urgent need for developing frameworks for practice that combine knowledge about trauma with the principles of anti-oppressive and emancipatory approaches. This theme aris-ing from my research resonates with the feminist and anti-oppressive range of theoretical approaches to practice (Adams *et al.*, 2009: 209–14).

As a result of repeating the development of the therapeutic relationship with each new client, the counsellor-participants drew from an eclectic mix of theories to inform their practice. Given the gross transgressions of physical boundaries that have taken place for the trauma survivor, the central dilemma for the therapist is, 'how can I supply what the cli-ent needs without replicating what happened before?' Second, 'if the occurrence of sexual abuse is indicative of skewed relationships in which power is misused and the survivor is denied her own subjectivity, how do I assist in the retrieval of the client's own voice?' The counsellor-participants' own training provided few constructive answers to these dilem-mas. Feminist approaches, theories that encompass principles of social justice and social systems, were found more useful. Frameworks that integrate the various strands of these theories (including the new trauma therapy) the counsellor-participants found to be the most relevant. Within the new trauma therapy the therapeutic relationship creates the climate in which clients can re-discover their own innate resilience and, through this awareness, can carry this knowledge into action in their everyday lives. The findings of my research sug-gest that there needs to be realignment in the philosophies of the funding organizations involved in sexual abuse work towards an approach consistent with these aims and with the practice of trauma therapists.

## Questions for reflection

- Overall, what is your impression of the comments made by the counsellor-participants? Do they 'ring true' to your own experiences?
- Which theories do you find most useful in your work, for example, trauma-informed theory, person-centred, narrative, psychodynamic theories of practice?
- How do these ideas (represented in these theoretical approaches used in your practice) fit within your own personal philosophy about why trauma such as abuse and domestic violence occur in society?
- Have your ideas about trauma and dealing with traumatic disclosures from clients changed or evolved over time with this understanding? How so? What are these changes?
- What experiences and events informed these changes in your belief systems over time?

## Case study 1: an example of how reference to a range of practice theories can inform practice with trauma survivors

The counsellor-participants used combinations of three main theoretical backgrounds that provided a framework for understanding the perspectives of their survivor clients. To begin with, narrative therapy overlaid with systems thinking that takes into consideration the socio-cultural and power dynamics underlying abuse within a patriarchal society was important to the counsellor-participants who were interviewed. Third, there was a spiritual dimension of holding the client's hope with the despair, which we will explore further in Chapter 8, that deals with spirituality and its relationship to therapist self-care. The privilege of hearing clients' stories of survival for the counsellor-participants interviewed was a source of inspiration and transcendence of the pain of witnessing. The notion of balance in dealing with and learning to hold both the client's despair and hope was considered crucial in this process. Hope is intrinsic to the work of psychotherapy yet it remains implicit in much of what we do as psychotherapists.

Sophia, a therapist who works in a feminist paradigm in the following excerpt from an interview for the vicarious traumatization study, refers to her experience of listening to stories of survival as enriching and 'expanding' her life, and at the same time, her 'tiredness':

> Sophia: It's changed me so much in terms of expanding my life. There are so many vicarious lives I have experienced now: not only vicarious trauma but also people's healing stories, just people's experiences and I feel like hearing so many people's healing stories, has broadened my experience bank enormously. That's a richness that is added in, a huge richness to my life. It's increased my tiredness, my patience and understanding and all sorts of things in a way that I find it hard to imagine any other field would do. I'm sure there would be, I guess, rewards in any service field or helping field and perhaps in many others too, but this one [trauma therapy] is particularly rich. Just knowledge about what it means to be human.
>
> [Pause to reflect] When I am sitting there hearing people's stories thinking: 'God, this is amazing!' That I am able to hear that story.

## Case study 2: the importance of hope in trauma-related therapy: a gestalt perspective

The concept of hope is discussed as I reflect upon an example from my practice that involves themes of vicarious traumatization and resilience. This case example begins with a description of the wider field of the community in which I worked to illustrate an approach to balancing hope and despair with my work with clients who were multiply abused (Pack, 2007). In situations of apparent 'no hope' illustrated in my practice with a middle-aged woman, a trauma survivor, and her family, I draw upon the underlying optimism and perseverance in gestalt therapy as the key to staying present and in the moment with the client. The underlying optimism and courage of gestalt theory, when operationalized, I conclude, is a vital component of clinician effectiveness and self-care when working therapeutically. In particular, hope and an attitude of 'optimistic perseverance' (Medeiros and Prochaska, 1988) are essential when working with clients who are living in situations of material deprivation and trauma, and whose presentation raises complex, existential themes and dilemmas for the therapist.

In 2005–6 I worked alongside the general medical practitioners at three suburban medical practices. These general practitioners' patients are amongst the lowest-income earners in suburban New Zealand. My brief in this community was to establish and provide with a small team a confidential and free mental health service that improved the access to service for residents who could not afford to use private services and yet did not fit the criteria for eligibility to the hospital mental health services.

As a high proportion of our clients were Māori and Pacific Islanders, but did not have ready access to culturally appropriate services, our 'Well-being' service comprised a *kaiawhina*, a registered nurse who works with traditional Māori healing methods, and a Pacific Peoples counsellor, fluent in two Pacific Island languages and cultures who used narratives from Pacifica to heal. The practice employed two advocates: a *kai-mahi* for Māori and a *matai* from Western Samoa, who helped families experiencing financial hardship to obtain the housing and benefits they needed to live.

As two rival gangs have headquarters in the region, domestic and gang violence was an everyday reality. Hope and courage were essential qualities in our relationships as colleagues working alongside residents of this community. As a team we were committed to engaging with one another and with our clients to 're-moralise', which according to Frank (2002) is possible through the quality of our relationships we have with one another. In this aim, we were drawing from Buber's (1970) notion of 'I–Thou' and what it means to be human which, for me, is the foundational idea in gestalt theory and practice. Buber's idea of being with the other in solidarity within which moments of being in connection arise spontaneously, creates the context within which the process of healing and 're-moralisation' (Frank, 2002) can begin.

In this section of the chapter, I draw material from my work with clients who bring to me their hope and despair about their life circumstances and I describe how I balance their hope and despair now that gestalt theory is informing my practice. On the surface, the concepts of hope and despair appear polarized or paradoxical. However, in working with them in complex situations, they become a gestalt. I will draw from the literature on vicarious traumatization (Pearlman and Saakvitne, 1995) and compassion fatigue (Figley, 1995) to suggest that gestalt psychotherapy contains the tools to stay well in engaging with materially deprived and traumatized clients. In particular, I will refer to the work of various gestalt therapists and theories that have inspired my optimism in gestalt theory as a guide to my practice in this setting. I will suggest that aspects of gestalt therapy can be used fruitfully to ameliorate vicarious traumatization.

I use the term 'gestalt theory' to refer to the core concepts underlying my practice. These concepts such as field theory (Parlett and Lee, 2005), the paradoxical theory of change (Beisser, 1970), the dialogical relationship (Hycner and Jacobs, 1995) and embodied practice (Kepner, 2003b) to my way of thinking are all part of the same gestalt as they are grounded in practice and they inform theory in their operation. Therefore, for me they are two parts of the whole. In this way, I conceptualize gestalt theory as both informing and enhancing practice with learning from my practice impacting upon and influencing what I do in an action–reflection process. I see the bridge between gestalt theory and practice as being Buber's (1970) conceptualization of 'I–Thou' as it is through the quality of relating and of the process of being in relationship from which all gestalt theory and therapy originates.

## Background

In the first two months of commencing work in this community, my personal belongings were stolen from the workplace and I witnessed a violent assault between a group of youths outside the rooms which provoked me to make an emergency call to the police. From this time, trust and safety issues became a day-to-day reality. I began to lock my possessions away every day in my filing cabinet as was the suggestion from the police. I was aware of feeling traumatized by the lack of security and control I was experiencing in my work environment.

The exposure to client narratives in this context had heightened my sense of vulnerability and fear of loss of control in the world. In retrospect I was over-identifying with client narratives. I was travelling a parallel path to the traumatized clients to whom I had been listening. I was so confluent with clients that I failed to maintain awareness of my own process while empathetically engaging with the client. To cope with the weight of traumatic disclosure, I was alternately merging with and distancing myself from the angst in the field created between us. As Zinker (1977) and many of the authors of the vicarious traumatization literature (Fox and Cooper, 1998; Pearlman and MacIan, 1995; Pearlman and Saakvitne, 1995; Pearlman *et al*., 1996) point out, this is a dangerous over-identification as it robs the therapist of her own space in which to process material brought to her from clients.

## Disruptions to the self and identity of the therapist: linkages to the literature on 'vicarious traumatization'

I believe that in gestalt psychotherapy, the support of colleagues assists the therapist to maintain a sense of connection to self and others and so remain 'contactful' (Clarkson, 2004; Joyce and Sills, 2001). Furthermore, it is participation in a professional community that enables therapists to connect to and embody their practice as a way of being (Kepner, 2003b). My experience is that connectedness enables me to both engage empathetically with the client's trauma, to recognize the parallel process of dissociation I sometimes experience in relation to traumatized clients and to recover from the 'contagion of dissociation' (Herman, 1992) and thus to be more present with the client.

## Therapist self-care

The literature on therapist resiliency and self-care assisted me to understand what I was witnessing in engaging empathetically in client narratives of deprivation, abuse and depression and the impact of these narratives on me. Disconnection with oneself, with one's family and friends and colleagues produces a sense of disjuncture that is the hallmark of vicarious traumatization (Pearlman and Saakvitne, 1995; Pearlman *et al*., 1996). I had noted this theme in researching the experience of sexual abuse therapists and their significant others in the New Zealand context (Pack, 2004). After experiencing periods of such disjuncture, I now valued and proactively used my own clinical supervision, personal therapy, social networks and sense of humour to increase my resilience to vicarious traumatization.

## A story of practice: Elizabeth

The case that has inspired this reflection on my practice is one of the most hopeful and the most vicariously traumatizing in my 20-year history as a mental health social worker and therapist. The client, Elizabeth Jones (pseudonym) was referred to the Well-being service by her general practitioner with a diagnosis of clinical depression. Thirty-nine-year-old Elizabeth, daughter of Bob, married and a mother of two children, had been supporting her parents throughout the long struggle of her father's depression. The Jones family had been referred earlier by the local crisis psychiatric team as their father, Bob, had been hospitalized during a suicide attempt that had nearly ended his life. This was Bob's sixth attempt at suicide. Elizabeth had resuscitated her father while waiting for ambulance assistance on one occasion.

On this occasion, the overdose of anti-depressants had left her father on life support systems. The family had asked the medical staff to turn the life support systems off as their understanding was that there was damage to the brain stem and the extent of his recovery was unknown. The family wished for his suffering to be over as they had witnessed his desire to end his own life since his unemployment in the late 1980s following an accident that left him in chronic pain with a back injury. While surviving on welfare payments for many years, he was assessed as fit to return to work but could not find work and became chronically depressed and suicidal from that point onwards.

What I experienced as traumatizing in this situation was that the family wanted the life support systems switched off and had lost all hope of recovery through what I assessed as compassion fatigue or vicarious traumatization. I found it difficult to support their decision due to strong beliefs I hold about the preciousness of life and because his prognosis was still unclear to the medical professionals. Thus, I was still holding out some hope of recovery for Bob and the family. While Elizabeth's presenting issue was clinical depression, I was also aware of taking a field theoretical position, or systemic position, in understanding my client in the context of her wider family issues.

The clinical specialists would not agree to switch off life support due to medico-legal ethical dilemmas so would not agree to the family's wishes. Elizabeth and her mother were planning to give up their employment to care full-time for their father/husband. This impending loss of employment and the prospect of full-time caregiving for Elizabeth and her mother seemed to add to and to compound the family's anguish which I found painful (though understandable) to observe (Pack, 2007 and Pack, 2009b).

## My responses to working with Elizabeth

In my individual sessions with Elizabeth, I began having physical responses in her presence. I wondered if there was something too awful for her to express. I experienced this response as a tightness in my solar plexus area that resulted in a kind of 'dread-filled' feeling when I sat with Elizabeth, noticing her smiling, dissociated face talking about her father's progress (or lack of progress) over the week. I hypothesized that she was suffering from PTSD that limited her range of affect to her frozen, smiling demeanour that greeted me on a weekly basis. Also informing my practice was my experience in relation to the client. I experienced anxiety, anger and powerlessness that I further hypothesized may have been denied or repressed by Elizabeth. Becoming acquainted with Jacobs's (2007) conceptual framework for understanding the psychological sequelae of trauma as being the event and the disruptions to subjective experience, 'TSM (traumatic states of mind or traumatic states of being)' resonated with what I was experiencing with Elizabeth. The hallmarks of 'traumatic states of being' (Jacobs, 2007), such as the loss of complexity of emotion, the past being contemporaneously experienced in the present with the client being triggered into organizing her world around survival, were themes in my contact with Elizabeth. The predominant feelings I experienced in relation to the client were dread and despair, mirroring the intensity of her anguish of living with a shattered world that had compounded over many years.

At this point, Elizabeth brought me a gift of chocolates to thank me, which added to my guilt at secretly wishing her father would recover. I believe I had supported her position (to turn the life support systems off), and I imagine she felt supported. This may have been because I had bracketed my responses to the life-versus-death decision that the family were facing. I found it difficult to support the decision of Elizabeth and her family as I felt that their decision was giving up on Bob. Giving up is not an option in my world view until death intervenes and connection (at least in this realm of existence) is then only possible among the living and the memory of the person who has died. At the same time my sense was that Elizabeth was more optimistic about the future and I felt that I was helping her through the crisis by listening empathetically to her narrative and supporting her decision to switch the life support systems off. I experienced my own rejection of the family's wishes and my guilt about having a different view and desired outcome. I knew that if I offered hope that this was important to the family, so I did not challenge their idealization of me as 'the helper' but privately I felt like a fraud.

I believed, as Clarkson (2004: 117) does, that it is an 'error' to 'hand back to clients' their idealized view of the therapist too early in therapy, in case it deprives them of hope. My sense was that I needed to have the courage to tolerate the ambiguity and complexity of the situation and what might happen to allow the family to define the way forward in their discussions with the medical professionals. I felt that I needed to acknowledge Beisser's (1970) paradoxical theory of change: that within each individual there is a uniquely individual theory of change awaiting discovery. I felt that I needed to explore with Elizabeth what her theory of change was by attending to her in the present moment.

## 'Optimistic perseverance': applications of gestalt theory

Gestalt theory was helpful in untangling this paradox of hope and despair in my practice with the family, and in understanding transference and countertransference phenomena. Kepner (1987, 2003a) discusses countertransference responses or the co-created field between the therapist and the trauma survivor as affecting the body of the therapist. Clients are frequently triggered into traumatized states by current events within the therapeutic relationship which often mirror themes from the past. It is not uncommon for the therapist to take these repressed or denied feelings to supervision to be understood and worked through due to their having a symbolic representation in the field of the therapeutic relationship (Kepner, 1987).

To understand my reactions to the client, I referred to the bodily signs that had become familiar to me over the weeks to 'track' my process with Elizabeth with my clinical supervisor. I became aware that my sense of dread became more tolerable as I built enough rapport with Elizabeth to be able to lean towards the meaning she was making from the tragic events surrounding her father's life. This approach enabled me to 'optimistically persevere' (Medeiros and Prochaska, 1988) to support Elizabeth, out of which more insights came. I reflected to her that living under the constant reality of seeing her father suffer with his depression might inspire a fear that she might follow a similar path. Articulating this unspoken fear for the client opened the floodgates to grieving for a loss of her hope for herself, in the face of her own depression linked to her father's recent suicide attempt.

This was the 'creative process' Zinker (1977) refers to in his suggestion of staying with the client's uncertainty until there is a creative insight and a time to offer this to the client: I wondered how she had lived with such a high level of despair for most of her adult life and I reflected upon the heroism of her struggle. Zinker suggests that 'a sense of wonderment' enables therapists to experience the special or unique qualities of their clients. He proposes that 'by staying with the situation, no matter how difficult, many factors emerge'. The skill of the 'creative' therapist is to 'track' these themes 'to maintain a sense of thematic direction', and to avoid becoming overwhelmed by the client's despair (Zinker, 1977: 47). In my view, the skill is to have confidence in the relational process and my part within it so that I know that through my own self-awareness there is a regulatory process in place that protects us both. It is through self-awareness that I can know also when I am becoming overwhelmed by despair triggered by my empathetic engagement in the client's story of tragedy and to recover from it more quickly to be more available to her.

As I continued to persevere optimistically, I was able to track the source of the client's own traumatization. In the course of sessions, Elizabeth disclosed that she and her siblings had been sexually abused by a close family member over many years. Her father had confronted the alleged perpetrator but this disclosure was met with denial. Her process of dissociation was a way of protecting herself both from this denial and from the flashbacks of abuse over many years. As Kepner (1987: 20) suggests, 'when the truth of violation is denied, the solution is to detach from her body and "its" reality'. Her previous four years of therapy had been of some assistance in healing from the aftermath of childhood sexual abuse, but the damage from her experiences was ever-present and to a large extent, expressed non-verbally. The co-created field of our experience picked up on these memory traces which I noticed as principally bodily responses. Through her anger at her father's recovery, she began to access some of her body awareness. For the first time, she confronted her father's clinicians about the lack of preparation and follow-up services for his discharge from hospital. She appeared animated and more alive.

I reflected to her the enlivening process that proceeded as she took charge to coordinate her father's care at home. The depression she had been experiencing lifted as she moved into a more powerful and active mode of self-expression. I witnessed and reflected to her what I noticed about her process – that, through the vehicle of anger, she appeared to be liberating herself from depression. My dread-filled responses dissipated. I theorized that the vicarious traumatization I had been experiencing diminished as increasing hope balanced the earlier despair.

## Conclusion

For me this case is an example of the 'creative process' (Zinker, 1977) possible in gestalt therapy whilst simultaneously illustrating the path through vicarious traumatization. By staying with the client's process, the present and what is, however grim, I was able to hold on to my own sense of hope. In an 'I–Thou' moment in relationship with Elizabeth, I had an insight of a paradox or polarity in my practice: that when I am working with despair and tragedy, that hope is also present in the field. Balancing my own hope and despair and the client's hope and despair, enabled me to stay more present with her. Elizabeth was able to use this space created between us to access more of her own feelings to interact with her environment and so to ask to have her needs met.

I also learned that the more I am aware of the need of some clients to organize their lives around trauma and survival, the more I am able to understand their process. When Elizabeth's coping façade was lowered due to fatigue in the caregiving role, I could more easily see how her original trauma (childhood abuse), compounded with subsequent traumatic events (her father's accident, injury, unemployment and depression), existed alongside the triggering of accommodation strategies to the original traumatic event. In my attempts to navigate the complexity of engaging empathetically with the client's process following years of traumatization, I was aware of a connection with an unspoken and intense mixture of feelings that translate most accurately as despair.

For me, the feelings evoked were accompanied by a physical sense of dread. Paradoxically, the more able I was to recover from my own discomfort with the feelings evoked in my experience in this empathetic engagement, the more easily I was able to tolerate ambiguity and to hold on to the uncertainty of travelling this path with compassion. I believe the willingness to be in solidarity with the client to undertake a search for meaning to attach to their experience is the part that truly heals. The client's awareness of my solidarity with her in this mutual search for meaning supports the possibility that another version of events exists even if it is only a glimmer in the distance.

To my way of thinking, my practice with Elizabeth is an example of paradox and of the paradoxical theory of change (Beisser, 1970) in action. The process of holding hope and despair, my own and that brought to me by Elizabeth, formed a complete gestalt. Maintaining an awareness of my own process and untangling the apparent paradox of hope and despair freed me from over-identifying with the client to risk travelling again the path of vicarious traumatization. This path, once feared, is now well known, well trod and successfully traversed.

## References

ACC. (2015). *ACC register of approved counsellors*. Retrieved from www.acc.co.nz/making-a-claim/ what-support-can-i-get/registered-counsellors/index.htm (accessed 28 February 2016). *Responding to ACC tenders*. Retrieved from: www.acc.co.nz/PRD_EXT_CSMP/groups/external_providers/ documents/guide/wpc118352.pdf (accessed 28 February 2016).

Adams, R., Dominelli, L. and Payne, M. (2009). *Critical practice in social work*. Basingstoke: Palgrave Macmillan.

Badger, K., Royse, D. and Craig, C. (2008). Hospital social workers and indirect trauma exposure: An exploratory study of contributing factors. *Health and Social Work, 33* (1), 63–71.

Bass, E. and Davis, L. (1988). The Courage to Heal: A guide for women survivors of child sexual abuse. New York: Harper and Row.

Beisser, A. (1970). The paradoxical theory of change. In Fagan, J. and Shepherd, I. (Eds). *Gestalt therapy now* (pp. 77–80). Palo Alto, CA: Science and Behaviour.

Briere, J. (1996). *Therapy for adults molested as children: Beyond survival*. New York: Springer.

Buber, M. (1970). *I and Thou*. New York: Charles Scribner's Sons.

Clarkson, P. (2004). *Gestalt counselling in action*. London: SAGE.

Coffey, R. (1998). *Unspeakable truths and happy endings: Human cruelty and the new trauma therapy*. New York: Sidran Press.

Courtois, C. A. (1997). Healing the incest wound: A treatment update with attention to recovered memory issues. *American Journal of Psychotherapy, 51* (4), 464–97.

Dalenberg, C. (2000). *Countertransference and the treatment of trauma*. La Jolla, CA: American Psychological Association.

Davis, L. and Bass, E. (1992). *The courage to heal* (3rd edn). New York: Harper Perennial.

Figley, C. R. (Ed.). (1995). *Compassion fatigue: Secondary traumatic stress disorder from treating the traumatised*. New York: Brunner/Mazel.

Fook, J., Ryan, M. and Hawkins, L. (2000). *Professional expertise: Practice, theory and education for working in uncertainty*. London: Whiting & Birch.

Fox, R. and Cooper, M. (1998). The effects of suicide on the private practitioner: A professional and personal perspective. *Clinical Social Work Journal, 26* (2), 143–57.

Frank, A. W. (2002). Relations of caring: Demoralisation and remoralisation in the clinic. *International Journal for Human Caring, 6* (2), 13–19.

Freire, P. (1970). *Pedagogy of the oppressed* (M. Bergman Ramos, Trans.). New York: Seabury.

Geertz, C. (1975). *The interpretation of cultures: Selected essays*. London: Basic Books.

Gelso, C. J. and Hayes, J. A. (2007). *Countertransference and the therapists' inner experience: Perils and possibilities*. Mahwah, NJ: Lawrence Erlbaum.

Hayward, J. (2009). Letter to the editor. *Listener*, October 17, pp. 6–7.

Herman, J. (1992). *Trauma and recovery*. New York: Basic Books.

Hycner, R. and Jacobs, L. (1995). *The healing relationship in gestalt therapy: A dialogic/self psychology approach*. New York: Gestalt Journal Press.

Jacobs, L. (2007). Pacific Gestalt Institute's winter retreat lecture (audiotape). Santa Barbara, CA.

Joyce, P. and Sills, C. (2001). *Skills in gestalt counselling and psychotherapy*. London: SAGE.

Kay, M. (2009). Review of sex abuse compo: New rules for ACC claims to be checked in 6 months. *Dominion Post*, October 28, p. A-2.

Kepner, J. I. (1987). *Body process: Working with the body in psychotherapy*. San Francisco, CA: Jossey-Bass.

Kepner, J. I. (2003a). *Healing tasks: Psychotherapy with adult survivors of childhood abuse*. Cambridge, MA: Gestalt Institute Press.

Kepner, J. I. (2003b). The embodied field. *British Gestalt Journal, 12* (1), 6–14.

McCann, I. L. and Pearlman, L. A. (1990). Vicarious traumatisation: A framework for understanding the psychological effects of working with victims. *Journal of Traumatic Stress, 3* (1), 131–49.

Medeiros, M. E. and Prochaska, J. O. (1988). Coping strategies that psychotherapists use in working with stressful clients. *Professional Psychology: Research and Practice, 19* (1), 112–14.

Pack, M. J. (2004). Sexual abuse counsellors' responses to stress and trauma: A social work perspective. *New Zealand Journal of Counselling, 25* (2), 1–17.

Pack, M. (2007). The concept of hope in gestalt therapy: Its usefulness for ameliorating vicarious traumatisation. *Gestalt Journal of Australia and New Zealand, 3* (2), 59–71.

Pack, M. (2009a). Revisions to the therapeutic relationship: A qualitative inquiry into sexual abuse therapists' theories for practice as a mitigating factor in vicarious traumatisation. *Aotearoa New Zealand Social Work Review, 21/22* (4/1), 73–82.

Pack, M. (2009b). Social Work (Adult). In Grimmer-somers, K. and Nehrenz, G. (Eds). *Practical Tips In Finding the Evidence: An Allied Health Primer* (pp. 176–199). Manila, Philippines: UST Publishing House.

Pack, M. J. (2010a). Transformation in progress: The effects of trauma on the significant others of sexual abuse therapists. *Qualitative Social Work: Research and Practice, 9* (2), 249–65.

Pack, M. (2010b). Career themes in the lives of sexual abuse counsellors. *New Zealand Journal of Counselling, 30* (2), 75–92.

Pack, M. (2014). Vicarious resilience: A multilayered model of stress and trauma. *Affilia: Journal of Women and Social Work, 29* (1), 18–29. doi: 10.1177/0886109913510088

Parlett, M. and Lee, R. G. (2005). Contemporary gestalt therapy: Field theory. In Woldt, A. and Toman, S. (Eds). *Gestalt therapy: History, theory and practice* (pp. 41–63). London: SAGE.

Pearlman, L. A. and MacIan, P. S. (1995). Vicarious traumatisation: An empirical study of the effects of trauma work on trauma therapists. *Professional Psychology: Research and Practice, 26* (6), 558–65.

Pearlman, L. A. and Saakvitne, K. W. (1995). *Trauma and the therapist: Countertransference and vicarious traumatisation in psychotherapy with incest survivors*. New York: Norton.

Pearlman, L. A., Saakvitne, K. W. and staff of the Traumatic Stress Institute. (1996). *Transforming the pain: A workbook on vicarious traumatisation for helping professionals who work with traumatised clients*. New York: Norton.

Reason, P. (Ed.). (1988). *Human inquiry in action: Developments in new paradigm research*. London: SAGE.

Reinharz, S. (1992). *Feminist methods in social research*. New York: Oxford University Press.

Shuttleworth, K. (2012). ACC making little progress on sensitive claims report. *New Zealand Herald*, July 17. Retrieved from www.nzherald.co.nz/nz/news/article.cfm?c_id=1&objectid=10820174 (accessed 28 February 2016).

Steed, L. G. and Downing, R. (1998). A phenomenological study of vicarious traumatisation amongst psychologists and professional counsellors working in the field of sexual abuse/assault. *Australasian Journal of Disaster and Trauma Studies, 1998* (2). Retrieved from www.massey.ac.nz/~trauma/issues/1998-2/steed.htm (accessed 28 February 2016).

White, M. (1997). *Narratives of therapists' lives*. Adelaide: Dulwich Centre Publications.

Yin, R. (1985). *Case study research*. New York: SAGE.

Zinker, J. (1977) *Creative process in gestalt psychotherapy*. New York: Vintage Books.

## Further reading

Dutton, M. A. (1992). *Empowering and healing the battered woman: A model for assessment and intervention*. New York: Springer.

Follette, V. M., Polusny, M. and Milbeck, K. (1994). Mental health and law enforcement professionals: Trauma history, psychological symptoms, and the impact of providing services to child sexual abuse survivors. *Professional Psychology: Research and Practice*, *25* (3), 275–82.

Grosch, W. N. and Olsen, D. C. (1994). *When helping starts to hurt: A new look at burnout among psychotherapists*. New York: Norton.

McCarroll, J. E., Blank, A. S. and Hill, K. (1995). Working with traumatic material: Effects on Holocaust Memorial Museum staff. *American Journal of Orthopsychiatry*, *1* (1), 66–74.

MacGibbon, J. (Ed.). (1978). *Stevie Smith: Selected poems*. Harmondsworth: Penguin Books.

Martin, C. A., McKean, H. E. and Veltkamp, L. J. (1986). Post traumatic stress disorder in police working with victims: A pilot study. *Journal of Police Science and Administration*, *14* (2), 98–101.

Melnick, J. and Nevis, S. M. (2005). The willing suspension of disbelief: Optimism. *Gestalt Review*, *9* (1), 10–26.

Moulden, H. M. and Firestone, P. (2007). Vicarious traumatisation: The impact on therapists who work with sexual offenders. *Trauma, Violence and Abuse*, *8* (1), 67–83.

# Chapter 3    **Developing new meanings for practice**

## Back from the edge of the world

My approach to therapy 20 years ago I am pleased to say that it is very different to what it is now. I betray my age by a Bob Dylan line: 'I was so much older then I'm younger than that now' [audience laughs].

There is more of a tentativeness in how we [client and therapist] unfold the session. I am very interested in memories – in autobiographical memories and giving people a chance to tell their story and unfold that. But I come from a background of cognitive-behavioural therapy and I can see that there are a lot of powerful procedures in that approach that I incorporate. So a lot of my therapy is balancing that idea, that getting the person's life and story with these interventions.

*Professor Glen Bates (2006) discusses his reformulated approach to therapy at the 'Roundtable' preceding the Gestalt Australia and New Zealand Conference, Melbourne, Australia*

## Introduction

In this chapter, building on the perspectives of the therapists I had earlier interviewed, who remained working as trauma therapists for many years, we begin to explore the notion of therapist resilience in the face of trauma with reference to the research literature. As the quote from the therapist above suggests, this understanding about how to most effectively and respectfully engage and work with clients therapeutically builds over time, with experience. Pieces of earlier training, though useful, are assessed for relevance continually, and are combed for new directions as the number of clients the therapist sees grows, and expertise and knowledge expand in the field. In this process, parts of one's earlier training may seem less relevant or appropriate and are gleaned for new directions (Pack, 2004, 2010). Original models and interventions in which we are trained may not be as applicable as whole frameworks, therefore, where found less applicable, these are adapted and modified with other approaches. This theoretical eclecticism was a feature of the trauma therapists' approaches whom I had earlier interviewed. Reference to an array of theories is a recommended way of approaching and working with trauma where a one-size-fits-all approach is generally considered less helpful to understanding the effects of complex trauma and the healing process following traumatic events (Harms, 2015).

The comment above also highlights another important learning reiterated by the counsellor-participants: that flexibility, humour, and balance and adaptation all assist therapists to deal with the many difficult emotional responses they face in dealing with traumatic material from their clients. I was again prompted to consider: what factors and personality traits enable some trauma therapists to persist and in fact thrive in their careers compared to others who decide to leave the field or the profession through experiences of vicarious traumatization, compassion fatigue and burnout? Literature from psychology, psychotherapy and counselling research seemed to offer some guidance on the hardiness of therapists to withstand the rigours of the work. This literature, mentioned in Chapter 2 in overview, focuses on the notion of resilience, by which trauma therapists actively evolve new meanings about their work and life while balancing hope with despair (Figley, 2006).

## Resilience

Recent research has suggested that the ability to 'bounce back' after traumatic experiences is more common than originally envisaged (Harms, 2015). For example, Bonnano (2004) and colleagues have researched different populations who had encountered traumatic and life-threatening events to conclude that around one-third of all of the populations surveyed did so without any formal psychological intervention. The factors that assisted individuals to successfully adapt following bereavement and post-traumatic stress involved their accessing their social networks to gain support and to avoid isolation (Bonnano, 2004). Withdrawal is a common response to stress, grief and trauma as well as being a hallmark of vicarious traumatization (Pearlman and Saakvitne, 1995). Being able to use relationship to evolve new meaning for the future is intimately connected with the capacity to experience and sustain a range of negative and positive emotions about trauma work (Collins, 2008a, 2008b). These emotional competencies are seen among those who successfully come through traumatic experience without long-term effects such as depression and anxiety (Bonnano, 2004). For professionals dealing with vicarious traumatization, social isolation is seen as both a sign of and a risk factor compounding the problem. Conversely, seeking peer review, consultation and clinical supervision is seen as being a protective factor to developing permanent ongoing negative responses from the nature of the work (Cunningham, 2003). The role of personal as well as professional support is a continuing theme in the literature on promoting self-care for helping professionals (Collins and Long, 2003). Whether this support is on a one-to-one basis, in groups or involving whole communities as occurs during professional conferences is a matter for the individual therapist to decide in relation to which supports are helpful. Assessment of support needs relies in turn on the trauma therapist remaining sensitive to his or her own personal biography and what is culturally appropriate for the individual.

Positive responses, optimism and hope have also been associated with the capacity to rebound through empathetic engagement with traumatic disclosures as a therapist. Optimism in the context of professional helping has been defined as being able to appraise situations positively and pro-actively, evolving coping strategies within the usual difficulties and complexities of the nature of the work (Collins and Long, 2003). Trotter (1999) has emphasized the role of optimism in forging and maintaining effective therapeutic relationships with clients, which sits alongside therapists' capacity for empathy, humour and limited self-disclosure in the therapeutic relationship.

Inevitably, abuse and trauma therapy more generally involves a political analysis of power and powerlessness to explain the prevalence of the victimization of vulnerable members such as women and children in society. How trauma therapists think through this analysis and integrate it into their personal and professional narrative is also relevant to the discussion about vicarious traumatization and what ameliorates it. This is what Parton and O'Byrne (2000) refer to as 'experienced optimism' or the positive belief about the potential of humankind to heal and transform various traumas and abuses over time. This knowledge forms a framework for understanding the healing process of those survivors whom therapists see daily in their practices.

Another protective factor involves the trauma therapists' capacity for critical reflection of their own practice. Deconstructing what is known relies on the therapist's self-awareness and draws from a variety of theoretical approaches as we saw the counsellor-participants doing in the previous chapter. These theories guiding the process of deconstructing the known include narrative, strengths-based, feminist, emancipatory and systemic therapies (Pack, 2010). Let's begin by focusing on narrative theories of practice to demonstrate how the use of narrative brings into a whole the memory fragmented by trauma and by vicarious traumatization.

## The role of narrative in healing from trauma

Narrative therapists Michael White and his co-author David Epston suggest that we can become enmeshed in 'dominant discourses' endorsed by the powerful groups in society that can disrupt our sense of 'personal agency' (White, 1995; White and Epston, 1990). When such a disjuncture between the life one wishes to live and the life others attribute to us exists, a common response is for individuals and families to seek help in the form of therapy.

Michael White developed his theoretical perspective about the usefulness of narrative in his therapy with clients after reviewing anthropological accounts of meaning-making across different cultural contexts. Drawing on the work of sociologists and anthropologists such as Geertz and Myerhoff provided the evidence-based practice on which to build his theories. The concept of *re-authoring* White (1997) developed derives from the work of anthropologists Turner, cited in Myerhoff (1982, 1992). Myerhoff, a cultural anthropologist and ethnographer lived among Jewish elders in her local community in Florida, while she completed an ethnographic study of Jewish elders. She writes of the sense of disjuncture that the Jewish elders experienced in migrating from the old country of Israel to the new country of America, having endured the horrors of the Holocaust. Drawing from extended narratives that began as conversations with Jewish elders at the community centre where they gathered for socializing and remembering the old country and Judaism, she describes the way that they tell and retell their personal biographies to integrate the traumatic memories with the good memories from the past. This narrative is one in which they describe escape from trauma, coming to a new life in America and the experience of growing old (Myerhoff, 1982). In this telling and retelling, she notices that their accounts are overlaid with the traditions, language and ritual of the old country. In reliving these experiences in the present, the process of 'remembering' is revealed to her. The term 'remembering' relates to a repopulating of family and friends once lost in space or time as elders are reunited with their significant others in the storytelling. New life-enhancing possibilities are created for the teller of the story in this 'remembering' as well as for the audience who interacts with the storyteller (Myerhoff, 1982).

This 'remembering' occurs in reflective or 'liminal spaces'. Myerhoff (1982) conceptualises liminal spaces as being holding places that exist between an old and familiar life and the new. This place is akin to the departure lounge at the airport where the old ways of being are no longer current, but can be reminisced about. The life to be can be imagined even though the new destination has yet to be arrived at. Liminal spaces offer a sanctuary for integrating the past, present and future ideas and thoughts about one's life story.

White conceptualizes 'remembering' as a process therapists may equally engage with as narratives of their own lives (White, 1997). The aim is to enable therapists to reconnect with lost or debased personal and practice narratives using the wisdom of community and significant others to repopulate and re-author lives (White, 1997). David, one of the counsellor-participants in the research I conducted, found narrative therapy, grounded in the work of White and Epston (1990), provided a means of using his own narrative about surviving traumatic experiences of bullying by a manager in the workplace. His own critical analysis of that situation was needed to assist clients who were dealing with similar challenges. David found his training as a clinical psychologist to be 'further abusive' and 'counter-therapeutic' in prescribing a purely clinical focus. He saw trawling through the minutiae of abuse recollections that was a requirement of reporting to statutory agencies for insurance cover on behalf of his clients as 'abusive'. As he moved into systemic and family therapies, he found he was able to re-author his own professional narrative as a therapist adapting his approach and earlier training as a clinical psychologist. Once he had felt alone, he repopulated his professional life with conferences with like-minded colleagues. A sense of community developed from his involvement with 'reflecting teams' who were involved in family therapy . He connected with colleagues who were interested in moving their practice to integrate narrative ideas and practices. As an interest group they used their involvement in reflecting teams to critically appraise their work and to relate theory to practice. For David this isolation he had experienced within the agency dissipated and his involvement with narrative and a community of trauma therapists who were interested in acting for one another as a 'reflecting team' ameliorated his experience of vicarious traumatization (Pack, 2010).

To illustrate the process of resilience in trauma therapists' work, I turn to the narrative of another of the counsellor-participants in the research I have conducted who uses her own narrative of survivorhood to act as a bedrock for her practice as a registered sexual abuse therapist. This case study of Carolyn demonstrates how resilience is prefaced on both holding hope for one's survivor clients as well as for oneself, concurrently. This allows a greater depth of engagement with clients whose narratives, at least initially in one's career, are hard to hear.

## Holding the hope for one's clients and oneself as therapist: Elizabeth's story of practice

Carolyn is self-employed in her own private practice after many years spent in senior managerial roles with a community counselling agency. Over the length of her career now in excess of 30 years, she saw structural and systemic approaches on their own as less meaningful to those theoretical approaches that involved clients' narratives about their lives. Over the years of her working career as a therapist she discussed changes in the ways in which she analysed structural inequality, power and powerlessness. With this expanded lens of analysis she increasingly viewed the connections between the personal and the professional. This perspective led her to reflect upon how she became involved in therapy herself which was at the outset fuelled by a desire to help parents who felt at risk of harming their children as a helpline volunteer in the 1970s. At this time, abuse of children was a topic not openly discussed. Carolyn listened regularly to a local radio programme where through talkback with other listeners, she began resonating with the experiences of the audience as herself a young mother of two children. She had experienced the difficulties of being at home with pre-schoolers, the loneliness and frustration associated with the role that was undervalued by society. Isolated incidents of parents hitting children as an act of discipline, however, were not seen at that time as a 'cry for help' as these parents' narratives were not disclosed for fear of negative judgement. Reflecting back on her own personal narrative, Carolyn acknowledged the role of her own parenting experiences as informing her decision to volunteer on the parenting telephone counselling service. As she listened to the stories of parenting from clients she was able to contextualize stories of trauma and abuse told and retold over the helpline. This holding of despair – her own and that encompassed in the stories she heard during her early experiences as a telephone counsellor – assisted her to develop more compassion and empathy for parents pushed to physically discipline their children. Often she heard mothers being abused themselves by partners and husbands, who were then hitting their children thus promoting a 'cycle of violence'. Initially this raised anti-male attitudes which she was constructively able to transform on the basis of the contextual issues heard in the narratives of parents:

> Carolyn: So then I moved into my aggressively 'anti-male mode'. All men were bastards, and while I have modified that quite a lot, I now don't automatically feel my hackles going up when any man opens his mouth. I still retain that clear analysis that men carry so much privilege that they are not aware of. The vast majority of them have absolutely no idea that they even have it [power], let alone how to manage it. But I am able to have more compassion for the fact that they don't notice it and so I just explore what I can do that might increase their awareness of it, especially their lack of awareness that it is stuffing up their lives all the time.

Carolyn had herself experienced abuse within her marriage which she had worked through with her own therapist. This autobiographical account of how she overcame the abuse in her marriage to go on to help other women was a source of wisdom she drew upon in her work with women survivors of sexual abuse in her private practice as she goes on to explain in the following excerpt from an interview for my research:

> Carolyn: If I were to tell, well I have told my life story heaps of times. My whole telling of my life story is based on choosing the language of the power of relationships and abuse of whatever sort. This features very strongly in the telling of my story and my children's story. Sexual abuse is one of the threads of it … that while the various abuses would have been better if they hadn't happened, the fact that they did has meant that the mission of my life has been to figure out what I do about it all. Whether it is for me personally, for my children or my clients, for my friends, for my colleagues. So my lenses that I use to look at the world are always abuse issues or power relationships.

## The power of narrative to address the impact of the intergenerational trauma of colonisation

Storytelling and narrative crosses cultural boundaries with yarning a common way for Aboriginal and indigenous people to integrate and make sense of everyday experience (Bacon, 2013: 136–65). Therapists who self-identified as Māori in the research on vicarious traumatization discussed how they drew upon their identity and position within Māoridom to restore and replenish. This theme was particularly striking for two of the counsellor-participants, Maxine and Linda, who both self-identified as Māori. Linda viewed the colonization of Aotearoa New Zealand by Pakeha settlers as a parallel process to abuse and violence, echoing the voice of writers such as Tuhiwai Smith (1999) who documents the connections between colonization and the loss of first peoples' stories. Colonization in this sense constitutes a kind of rape. Deconstructing the narratives underlying colonization is a way of breaking down Eurocentric accounts of 'history' to reveal the lived experience of first peoples whose stories have been rendered invisible, over centuries. The goal of therapy becomes one of helping people to access their stories through a conversation that can then be returned to the families who created them. Linda developed her thinking about the links between colonization and trauma as a consequence of exploring her cultural identify and what being Māori meant for her. This knowledge of herself as a woman from a lineage of Māori healers guided her practice with clients, most of whom also self-identify as Māori:

> Linda: As I have become more whole in terms of being a Māori woman, I've developed a bigger-picture understanding, too, of how this whole area of work relates to Māori in particular. Because, I work with Māori and I very rarely work with non-Māori ... the identity issue is really important. So if we just look at that it would be about people making contact with your *whānau* [extended family] and exploring their *whākāpapa* [genealogy] and finding out about where they come from and their particular *iwi* [tribal affiliation] and to be able to go home, being able to know where their *marae* [tribal meeting place] is and being involved in all that kind of stuff. But I also think the spiritual, being part of nature, building really good support networks, finding support for whatever direction they are wanting to take their life whether that be in terms of their education or career. Just that whole-picture thing really. All aspects of their lives is what is ultimately going to be the healing stuff.

Trauma therapists such as Linda and Maxine saw their role as therapists as assisting their clients to find and locate their identity as Māori within *whākāpapa* (genealogy), *whānau* (extended family), *hapū* (sub-tribe) and *iwi* (tribe). Through making these connections to their identity they located themselves within the stories of their living descendants as well as distant ancestors now in spirit. These ways of working nurture what Westerners refer to as 'spirituality' or those intangible aspects of everyday life that nurture the self and heal the fragmentation that is a feature of dealing with trauma. Linda and Maxine acknowledged that to be most effective with their clients they needed to reflect on their own sources of cultural replenishment and nurturance. Maxine enjoyed living for longer periods in the bush in a family cottage in a remote location where she was able to reconnect with the spiritual aspects of her being. She discovered that in natural surroundings where the environment inspired her inner journey of discovery she was able to maintain her wellness and professional effectiveness as a trauma therapist. Celebrating nature, community and belonging is among the key antidotes to vicarious traumatization (Pearlman and Saakvitne, 1995). We will explore this theme in more depth in Chapter 8 of this book.

## Locating oneself in a wider narrative: spirituality and belonging in community

Recurrent themes in discussions I had with the counsellor-participants involved seeing oneself as part of a connected universe of diverse beings. One therapist discussed a need to 'tread lightly on the soil', derived from a green vision of self-sufficiency and returning to the land for food and sustenance. In such discussions, the self is located in a sense of communal otherness that is primordial in origin, that exists beyond the confines of ego, time and place. This was described to me in various ways: as a 'sense of being', of 'presence' or 'oneness', 'transcendence', and of 'coming home to oneself'. Their significant others who were not working in the field of recovery from trauma and psychotherapy did not share this deeper reality and so were not expected by the therapists to understand them. Instead they told me stories of how they celebrated this appreciation of the everyday by documenting their experiences in professional conferences, in writing articles and commentaries for professional journals and in tweets from their webpages. They were recounting what Myerhoff describes in working with Holocaust victims in her ethnographic writings as 'a journey to the edge of the world of living' (Myerhoff, 1982: 25). This journey of finding a shared meaning with like-minded others following immersion in trauma is 'the survivor's return from that edge' (Myerhoff, 1982: 25). In a parallel way trauma therapists embark on a shared search for meaning that is akin to a journey back from the edge of the world. Being witness to the survivorhood of their clients, and in some cases their own survivorhood through vicarious traumatization, had served to 'intensify their dedication to social justice; they not only sought evidence of morality in a shattered, disordered world, but also worked to establish it' (Myerhoff, 1982: 25). These themes will be reported more fully in Chapter 8 when we explore the role of spirituality, nature and community in self-care.

To illustrate the value of constructing one's own narrative in practice with trauma survivors, I offer an ongoing reflection of the difficulties of working with trauma survivors within mental health agencies that provide brief models of intervention. The dilemma of how to work safely, respectfully and collaboratively with clients who present with a history of trauma is highlighted. As author of this narrative I reflect on my own experience of vicarious traumatization through my practice with a long-term survivor of domestic abuse. The team and organizational narratives that are embedded in the medical and managerial models in the mental health services are reflected upon as constraining the environment in which I attempt to provide a safe context for the client's healing and for collegial practice. By witnessing the abuse survivor's story of survival drawing upon themes in the 'new trauma therapy', gestalt and narrative therapy practice frameworks, I suggest that other versions of the 'story' are made available for the client and for the worker that offer a greater sense of 'personal agency'. These 're-authored' narratives offer a way forward for the client, individual worker and team (Pack, 2008).

Trauma is ameliorated when the retelling of a story is located within broad philosophic frameworks in which the whole person is attended to (Harms, 2015). Experience, both one's own and vicariously lived through listening to client accounts, needs to be located in perspectives that give meaning to experience in a holistic way. To illustrate this point, I offer the following critical reflection. This extended reflection explores, through my practice in a specific case of domestic violence, how I managed to evolve meaning to continue to cope with traumatic disclosures within the constraints of an agency. In my experience, this process was akin to a journey to the edge of the world. This example charts my return from the edge. This retelling of the story of my practice is put forward in the hope that others may benefit from these reflections. Articulating themes from practice provides another level of understanding. Out of such defining moments of practice new and reformulated frameworks for practice emerge.

In this case a synthesis is made connecting gestalt theories, based in holism and phenomenological methods, and narrative to describe the wider 'field' (Parlett and Lee, 2005) with narrative theory. This reflection explores how we can become enmeshed in 'dominant discourses' that are endorsed by powerful groups in society, which disrupt our sense of 'personal agency' (White, 1995; White and Epston, 1990). Narrative therapy is defined by White and Epston (1990: 121) as a process by which therapists 'work collaboratively with people in identifying those ways of speaking about their lives that contribute to a sense of personal agency, and that contribute to the experience of being an authority on one's life'. For White and Epston, therapy's aim is to assist people to recover lost narratives and wisdom that have been marginalized and debased by 'professional knowledges'.

## A narrative of my own practice

The following example from my own practice demonstrates a defining moment in my emerging professional identity as a psychotherapist (Pack, 2008). This narrative is based on my memory of pieces of work that were undertaken in my practice as a team leader of a mental health service I had established, while I was also training as a gestalt psychotherapy intern. This is a composite constructed out of a number of cases rather than one case. It contains themes and storylines that relate to 'vicarious traumatization' (Pearlman and Saakvitne, 1995), 'compassion fatigue' (Figley, 1995) and what ameliorates them. As suggested in previous chapters, these concepts refer to the process of self-transformation that occurs when the helper witnesses and engages empathetically with traumatic disclosures from clients. I also considered that it might demonstrate my praxis journey through my engaging in a critical-reflective process of a piece of my own work, in a way that is suggested in the writings of gestalt psychotherapists (Yalom, 1989; Zinker, 1977).

Looking back, I realized I had developed a quality of relationship with the client, Freda (not her real name), that went beyond my 'official' role as a mental health professional. Care in maintaining contact, trust and respect meant that I needed to go beyond the confines of 'the clinic', and notions of what is customary practice within the psychiatric or medical model. This way of working enabled Freda to trust me with more of her personal narrative, as time went on. However, my colleagues saw her presentations to the service where I was working over the course of a year as constituting 'a problem'. I wished to 'externalise the problem' (White, 1995) through the opportunity of retelling the story of my therapeutic relationship to Freda, and in that retelling, to re-author it. Returning to 'unfinished business' (Joyce and Sills, 2001) in an attempt to make a complete gestalt was another motivation to document this ongoing reflection.

I chose to focus on my practice in relation to one client who is a composite of many with whom I have worked, to avoid any breach of anonymity and confidentiality. A minimum of detail is included to tell this account of my practice. My working relationship with Freda, and many other woman clients in similar circumstances, illustrates the differing viewpoints and multiple, shifting realities that constitute accounts of practice. I refer to these accounts as 'stories' of practice because they reflect my reality of the events (Pack, 2008).

## Themes from working with survivors of abuse

Working for many years with sexual abuse survivors, I found that my initial training as a social worker provided few constructive answers to dilemmas involving maintaining relationships with those whose trust has been betrayed. Gestalt therapy with its emphasis on phenomenology, existentialism and holism, I discovered, was more useful than the psychoanalytic tradition from which social work (my original training) and psychiatry (the site of my work) drew. However, how to approach a new way of being with clients that separated me from my original training was difficult. I felt a little like Coffey (1998: 163) who concludes that 'therapists who toss aside all psychotherapeutic tradition may also unwittingly and perilously toss aside its protections, forcing themselves to blaze unnecessarily chancy paths through precarious jungles'.

There is an element of risk and of trailblazing through such 'jungles' that set me on the path of finding other ways of working with clients to ensure that their well-being and my own health was maintained in the process. The new trauma therapy epitomized in the work of Courtois (1988, 1997), Herman (1992), Briere (1996), Coffey (1998) and Dalenberg (2000) offered some initial ideas. Within such theories there is an emphasis on the therapist's own awareness of self and relationship to self and other that are the keys to maintaining connections with clients who have been traumatized. The 'blank screen' of Freudian psychoanalysis is replaced by a conceptualization of therapy as a collaborative endeavour in which the therapist is a witness who stands in solidarity with the client. Narrative and language are important in the healing journey of both the client and the therapist. With these themes in mind, I begin the story of Freda and our therapeutic relationship.

## My account of Freda's story

The local women's refuge referred Freda to the community mental health services where I was working as a psychiatric social worker. The refuge worker, who provided Freda with transport to our initial session, said that she had not been sleeping or eating well, and the workers were worried about her state of mind since her arrival there. The local women's refuge had provided emergency accommodation for Freda and her five children in the weeks immediately following a life-threatening assault by her husband after which he was arrested, convicted and imprisoned. Freda is a first-generation New Zealander whose parents had migrated to this country from China in search of a better life.

After the initial interview, I wrote and presented a bio-psychosocial assessment for presentation to the multidisciplinary team. The purpose of the assessment and the case presentation was to formulate a plan of action. The team agreed with my formulation that Freda seemed to be experiencing symptoms of clinical depression since the attack, and an appointment time was offered for her to see the consultant psychiatrist. The consultant psychiatrist confirmed the signs of depression I had noted in my assessment, prescribed medication and then referred Freda back to me for 'short-term counselling'. The expectation from the team was that I support Freda for six, weekly sessions to assist her to recover from the immediate crisis. The team thought that, in time, Freda would benefit from relaxation training to assist with her general level of anxiety stemming from PTSD. The assessment and treatment plan was implemented and Freda responded in a way that led to her discharge from our service.

However, she returned after the contracted six sessions. Freda did not fit the existing profiles of psychiatric services' client groups, who either had diagnosed long-term mental illnesses, and so justified longer-term care for those who were referred to as 'chronics' or for those needing shorter-term/acute services who were referred to as 'the worried well'. Brief models of intervention did not fit Freda's needs. The dilemma was that she appeared to have 'recovered' from the immediate crisis, was linked to community resources and, therefore, was no longer expected to need contact with mental health services.

She periodically returned to our community-based mental health centre once she had achieved some stability. This relative calm in her life that she cultivated in the weeks following her engagement with our service enabled her to remember further traumatic events that she had endured. Freda began to look at these themes in her family of origin in a number of ways. She joined a longer-term psychotherapy group and a community-based women's group that I had established in conjunction with the coordinator of a local women's centre. Looking back, these were attempts at contact and relationship when circumstances triggered a fixed gestalt from the past history of victimization within her marriage and family. My dilemma was that the team expected me to be the 'quick fix' change agent which conflicted with my understanding of the healing process for trauma survivors from a gestalt perspective (Kepner, 1987, 2003a, 2003b; MacKewn, 1997), narrative therapy (White and Epston, 1990; White, 1995) and earlier learning from the 'new trauma therapists' (Briere, 1996; Herman,

1992). My understanding was that listening to and engaging empathetically with the client and her narrative provides a space for 're-authoring' to proceed.

With this in mind, I return to my memories of my first meeting with Freda (Pack, 2008).

## Reflections on our first meeting and earlier contact

At the first meeting, I found Freda's presentation confusing. I found working with Freda overwhelming in the first contact, due to the weight of unexpressed, conflicting and con-tradictory emotions of which I was aware. I related these feelings, mistakenly in retrospect, to the latest attempt on her life. I realized, as our work together progressed, that the extent of the traumatization and her need for a different experience of relating were the probable reasons for her wish to re-present to our service.

My relationship with Freda, over the time in which I knew her, inspired many feelings, including revulsion at the way she had been treated, the anxiety that surrounded her day-to-day life, righteous anger towards her perpetrators and guilt/relief that I had been spared such horrors. I experienced the terror that went unexpressed by Freda and, at times, felt fearful that I, too, was at risk of violence by virtue of being a woman living in relationships and institutions based on patriarchal power dynamics.

Freda's survival became a source of wonderment to me, which I reflected to her. In the early months of our contact she discounted her resourcefulness. Eventually her desire was to take her driving test as a way of contributing to her growing independence.

## Major themes in the narrative of my practice

The metaphor of Freda wishing to be in the driver's seat of her own life became an enduring symbol of her growing independence, with the result that she took her driver's licence and purchased her own car. From this time onwards, I used the metaphor of Freda being in the driver's seat of her life. This goal created a context or 'experiential field' that made more available the process that I was interested in supporting (Kepner, 2003a). Her success at passing her driver's test foreshadowed her release from a marriage in which she had a 'spoilt identity' (White, 1995) attributed to her. White uses the term 'spoilt identity' to refer to the limited definitions of ourselves that we come to live by, through a process of internalization of what others call us. By the term 'spoilt identity', I refer to the tendency for Freda to make herself invisible as a means of coping with the domestic violence she had endured.

Through the use of metaphor, Freda created a vision of her future that differed from the images of her that were promoted by her interaction within her family of origin and with her own children. Our 're-authoring' involved inventing other versions of Freda and her story. Her car remained a potent symbol of her newfound sense of self that had been rendered invisible over 20 years of marriage. We drew upon the achievement of passing her driver's licence to challenge the versions of her story that were based in lack and in deficit. In retro-spect, the celebration and declaration of these new versions of her story, in line with White and Epston's (1990) work around performance and ritual in the presence of wider audiences, could have assisted in this 're-authoring'.

The public display of her car to the team, may have provided such a context in which her success was witnessed and celebrated by trusted others, albeit by her professional casework-ers. Experimentation with ceremony, ritual might have strengthened Freda's re-authoring of her narrative, as she had the paperwork to accompany her right to be in the driver's seat, via the attainment of her driver's licence. However, her personal narrative did not provide the scope at the time for acknowledging let alone celebrating such achievements.

## Reflections on my work with Freda

We looked at earlier events within Freda's family of origin as mirroring the events within her marriage. Freda was successful at changing her history by climbing back into the driver's seat of her life, despite invitations to remain firmly in the passenger's seat. My work with Freda involved listening to her stories, expressing wonderment at her endurance and persistence, working with her key desires and the metaphors they evoked. The stories Freda told to me supplied the *'sparkling facts'* and *'news of difference'* that seemed to spur her into upward cycles of success begetting success (White, 1995; White and Epston, 1990).

White and Epston (1990) use the terms 'sparkling facts' and 'news of difference' in the sense of being examples of exceptions to the predominant narrative that bring people to therapy. These narratives are often enmeshed with problems that relegate the client to an identity that is related to, or synonymous with, 'the problem'. To assist the person enmeshed in pathologizing discourses to gain space from being the problem, White and Epston encourage their clients to contemplate and recall the instances that fall outside the predominant discourse. They sometimes personify the problem that is threatening to take hold and give the problem a personal identity.

It was appropriate in my working with Freda to focus on the 'tellings and retellings' of her story as it brought into our awareness the possibility of working from other versions of the predominant story with which Freda had become identified and enmeshed.

## Theoretical underpinnings of my work with Freda

Such practice generates a process in which the client can recall and use skills and personal resources that have been obscured by the predominant narratives. From a gestalt perspective, the therapeutic relationship is the 'vehicle' of healing. As Kepner (2003b: 8) suggests:

> It is not our personality theory, nor our empty chairs or our creative techniques ... the core of what is healing in the Gestalt approach is our contextual, relational and experiential conditions that make for growth. It is the creation of a person/environmental field as the interactive whole in which growth may take place, just as it is the conditions of the field which create the 'mental health' problems which the client is bringing to us.

Sometimes it seemed important that I was simply there as a physical presence, to witness Freda experiment with her re-discovered abilities. Once Freda became familiar with her newfound talents, it became easier for her to access and use these abilities in her everyday life. Other trauma theorists have termed this process 'witnessing' (Dalenberg, 2000; Herman, 1992). I became the person who was the witness in the background until the process of integration of this knowledge of herself had been internalized. The importance of believing in Freda's talents and capabilities was the most foundational, guiding principle in my practice and continues to be so. From a gestalt perspective, if I lose the ability to see the resourcefulness that my clients bring along with the defined 'problem', I lack the frame of reference for forming a relationship in which the client can begin to have a different experience.

This work, given the history and transgressions of boundaries of the past, is of necessity carefully paced, evolving in slow, small, incremental steps. Becoming acquainted with Jacobs's (2007) conceptual framework for understanding the psychological sequelae of trauma as being the event and the disruptions to subjective experience, 'TSM (traumatic states of mind or traumatic states of being)' resonated with what I was experiencing with Freda. The hallmarks of 'traumatic states of being' (Jacobs, 2007) such as the loss of complexity of emotion, the past being contemporaneously experienced in the present with the client being triggered into organizing her world around survival, were themes in my contact with her.

## Pathologizing discourse in mental health

My experiences with Freda and other women, whom the team found complex, difficult and hard to reach, provided the impetus to find other options besides those offered within the confines of psychiatric services. In so doing, I became aware of the stigmatizing influence of being a client within an institutional/psychiatric setting. The problem was that I had engaged with a client who kept re-presenting which in itself constituted a 'problem' to the wider clinic. Such clients were often traumatized and so required longer-term care that was not, at that point in time, recognized within the wider mental health service. I wanted to provide an alternative pathway for clients who were in the process of healing from traumatic events, from a career as a 'psychiatric patient'. Due to Freda's numerous re-presentations at the outpatient clinic, the team I worked with suggested to me that I present my work with Freda at our monthly problem case conference.

## The 'problem' case conference

The focus of the therapeutic endeavour within the wider multidisciplinary team of psychiatric services in which I worked, assumed many forms. The hospital service offers individual psychological interventions, family therapy, nursing, psychiatric assessment and review; the provision of practical rehabilitation such as occupational therapy; the coordination of in-patient/community/day programme facilities; and social work. Re-integration into community life is the primary goal or outcome of contact, following hospitalization or treatment.

The provision of practical services such as advocacy to obtain income maintenance and housing is central to the multidisciplinary team's perceptions of the social worker's and so my role within the mental health service. As a qualified, experienced and registered social worker within the services that are primarily responsible for diagnosing and 'treating' clients, I was aware that I was also working as part of a system that, at times, seemed to be preventing clients from healing, despite my well intentioned efforts to the contrary.

My role primarily consisted of assessing and 'treating' clients. 'Treating' meant two-to-six sessions of individual or group sessions following initial assessment and the formulation of a treatment plan, by the team. This plan was a standard format detailing the presenting issue to the history and social circumstances of the client. The plan ended with a 'formulation' or summary that consisted of what the worker had surmised to be the key issues to be addressed. A range of services were then suggested, often in combination, with the intention of addressing the needs identified. What the plan lacked was a clear statement of what the client wanted, the absence of which led to the team unintentionally excluding the client from the development of the plan.

Such well-meaning efforts often involved the consumers of our service becoming what we referred to as 'chronics', who came and left the service in a revolving-door fashion. This group of longer-term clients was expected to spend varying amounts of time in contact with our services, so their presence did not constitute a 'problem' in the same way as Freda did. The clinic, or the context in which we worked defined, therefore, who or what was 'problematic'. Due to the challenges of such clients as Freda, the team implemented a monthly 'problem' case conference that all psychiatric staff in the greater area could attend, to deal with cases that were defined by the team as 'difficult'.

Much to my dismay, Freda had become known as a 'chronic' within psychiatric services. I felt blamed for failing to both reduce her re-presentations and demands on our service and for creating what the team implied was a dependence on me that could be thwarting her independence. Freda had refused to see any other staff member when she referred back to our service on a number of occasions. Over the year in which I knew Freda, she did, however, work with many different staff in a variety of roles, but would only see them after first seeing me. I became the first 'port of call' when she referred. As such, I was the one who then introduced different staff and team recommendations for Freda's consideration.

## Possible explanations for Freda's return

In retrospect, I could surmise the reasons for Freda's so called 'dependency' on me as her caseworker. From a client-centred perspective, my personal qualities, which could have been perceived by Freda as being consistency, dependability and trustworthiness, might have compensated for the disruption caused by trauma that she had experienced over many years. Freudian psychoanalysts might have concluded that I was a 'transitional person or object' while Freda reconstituted her life. The new trauma therapists (Briere, 1996; Herman, 1992) might have thought my approach in going at Freda's pace and dealing with practical skill-building before memory work, might have been deemed useful to Freda.

From a managerial viewpoint, I represented the whole of the multidisciplinary team in my person, and, therefore, the means of accessing a range of people and services and providing continuity of care. As Opie (2000: 5) suggests, as a representative of the multidisciplinary team, I provided 'the actual and conceptual point of intersection at which the multiple fragmented representations of the client's body are reassembled'. Narrative therapists might surmise that Freda was able to access alternative narratives in our sessions and, thus, re-author her personal story. As these new versions of her personal narrative became known to Freda and therefore accessible to her, I became the audience of one that witnessed Freda's performance of these alternative stories. My being witness to Freda's recounting and working from these alternative narratives might have led to the recovery of her stories and an enhanced sense of 'personal agency' (White and Epston, 1990: 17).

From a gestalt perspective, I could be seen as co-creating and holding a 'field' (Kepner, 2003a; Parlett and Lee, 2005) in which Freda was re-discovering her lost aspirations and dreams for the future. In this salvaging of her lost narratives through carefully attending to and supporting her process, her own resilience could have been recovered, the knowledge of which could then be integrated into her day-to-day life.

## 'Re-authoring' Freda's and my narratives: re-writing the way ahead

Freda and I both became immersed in pathologizing discourses (Hart, 1995; White, 1995). The team minimized Freda's achievements and she found herself labelled as a 'patient' within psychiatric services. Increasingly I began to be aware and uncomfortable about the structure in which I worked that seemed to appreciate neither the needs of traumatized clients such as Freda, nor the professional expertise that psychotherapy offers. What was a normal response to abnormal events in the case of domestic violence over many years became ensnared in psychiatric labels and discourse that added further injury to insult.

However, based on my gestalt training and personal awareness, I knew that to connect, and generate a field for supporting Freda's process into creating new ways of being, was one of the pathways to assisting her healing from trauma. Ironically, our service's failure to appreciate the needs of clients such as Freda seems to have been part of the reason why she and others regularly re-referred and became a 'problem' to our services. Unfortunately, I had experienced many clients who were recovering from trauma over my 20-year career in mental health who became labelled as 'depressed' which led on to a career in mental health services, often lasting some years.

## Reflections on team discourses

I reflected on the various discourses that had developed among my peers within the case conference. Through this kind of negative feedback, I began to doubt the skills and abilities I had developed as a fledgling gestalt therapist. I began to think I did not have a theoretical rationale for practice. Now, I recognize that the discourses I had been involved in while working in mental health had separated me from the basis of my practice, leaving me feeling disempowered and alienated from the theoretical grounding that had previously sustained and guided my work.

Part of the paradox was that not only was Freda typecast as a 'bad' or 'disobedient' client in child-like terms but, as the worker attached to her care, I was similarly stigmatized for creating and maintaining the 'problem'. The creation of pathologizing discourses surrounding me created a professional millstone around my neck from which I felt I could not escape until I left the service. Such conditions were conducive to creating a climate in which vicarious traumatization was very much a fact of my life and a daily reality. This experience inspired in me the need to find creative modes of liberation by looking at the wider 'field' including the team and the organizational context.

## Vicarious traumatization: a team perspective

In further contemplating the case study, I wondered if the interaction described among the multidisciplinary team reflected their collective and individual experiences of vicarious traumatization epitomized in a parallel process to the client's process. I considered the persistent search for additional services to 'fix' the problem that Freda represented. This was a discourse of vicarious traumatization in two senses. The first of these sources of vicarious traumatization is the wider organizational context in which the managerial 'time is money' ethos contrasted with the altruistic discourses of the team as an entity and as individual members. Both as individuals and as a team, it was not possible to provide the continuation of resources to support Freda's healing in her own time. Rather, goals, tasks and a desire to fix and discharge seemed to reflect the enmeshment and conflict among the team, individual and organizational discourses.

Opie (2000) argues for clarity in the face of wider organizational narratives where teams in similar situations and contexts are seen to constitute 'discourses of survival' and 'of failure'. Teams and individuals may take on other related discourses that are 'heroic', 'oppositional' or, if based in feelings of powerlessness, may defer to 'discourses of defeat'. According to Opie, the existence of multiple discourses grounded in multiple perspectives provides points of reference for teams and individuals to make meaning from their diverse experiences on the job. Opie recommends attending to the discourses at the individual, team and organizational levels in order to move out of the impasses caused by enmeshment in the more negatively framed discourses.

With the benefit of hindsight and the luxury of knowing what I know now, I return to reconsider my practice in relation to team discourses.

## 'Re-authoring' my practice

In retrospect, I could surmise that one possible reason for the team's impatience with Freda and the need to problematize her stemmed from the wider discourses of the hospital system and field at that time. As part of the wider psychiatric service, we were increasingly under pressure as individuals and as a team to collect statistics on client turnover, length of time of clients being in the system, and itemizing the use of our time on the job. The increasing managerialism that viewed public health as a commodity like any other in the business world might have conflicted with the altruistic ideals of individuals and teams working within mental health. The previous emphasis on client satisfaction was increasingly supplanted by efficiency, defined in terms of client turnover within specified time frames.

The vicarious traumatization that might have coalesced around the agendas of the wider organization of which we were all a part – to move clients swiftly through – produced 'discourses of failure', when our statistics were compared across other units within the hospital (Opie, 2000). 'Chronics' such as Freda came and left our service in a revolving-door fashion which was identified as problematic to the definition of an 'exit' to the service. Instead of remaining unspoken, these issues could have been collectively and openly discussed as informing our patterns of impatience with Freda. This would have changed our focus to what was happening within our agency rather than labelling the client with what was essentially our problem rather than hers.

## 'Re-authoring' the team narrative: the way ahead for clinicians

If I had been able to bring awareness to the group process to what was occurring within the multidisciplinary team, I could have reflected my own involvement in the discourse of failure that was not all my own making, although it felt like I was that discourse, at the time. Collectively, we could have discussed ways of responding to the gap between how we worked, both individually and as a team, alongside the wider organizational imperatives of economic retrenchment within the health services. We could have analysed the power differentials of the discourses we were espousing. The 'problem case conference' might then have been reformulated as narratives of individual survival and success despite various obstacles.

Stories of client resilience and worker or team creativity might have been discussed as engaging us in new discourses, some of which might have assumed a distinctly heroic appeal. We might then have been a team that invested time in exploring the wider organizational 'field' conditions that includes the environment of mental health workers, the clients, the team and the organization. The creation of a range of narratives within this 'field' of experience might have enabled our teams and individuals to author a range of narratives within the wider organization.

Having the space to choose one's own narrative among multiple discourses would have been a powerful mediator to the vicarious traumatization that I and no doubt others experienced individually and collectively within the team and wider organization at that time. The increased sense of *personal agency* (White and Epston, 1990) among the workers would then have been more likely to have flow-on effects to the quality of interaction with clients and co-workers in the workplace, in an upward rather than downward spiral.

## Conclusion: an awareness of 'dissonance'

Paradoxically, discussing this sense of disjuncture in working within a therapeutic relationship that lacks a fit between the service and the client's needs connects with the potential for exposure, shame and vicarious traumatization for the worker. In working with trauma, this dissociation can be a 'field' condition of working with sexual abuse and other traumatic disclosures in terms of the potential for vicarious traumatization and burnout that are routinely experienced on the job (Grosch and Olsen, 1994; Pearlman and MacIan, 1995; Pearlman, *et al.*, 1996). Shame and a parallel process is produced between the client and worker as 'victim' of a system that purports to care yet in its operation fails to promote the conditions for healing. It is best described as an experience of disconnectedness or dissonance.

Thus, dissonance occurs on two levels simultaneously: the discomfort of knowing that the work is outside the 'known' in the case of working with traumatic disclosures, coupled with working within a system that requires working in a way that challenges the need for a dialogic or collaborative relationship with clients.

In writing this reflection, I discovered creative ways of traversing the path 'back from the edge of the world'. Gestalt and narrative therapy are informing my practice now with trauma survivors. I am aware of the concepts of hope and despair in this reflection as being an apparent paradox or polarity on the surface. However, in working with them with traumatized clients in complex situations, they become a gestalt (Pack, 2008). Freda's depression could have been re-authored as demoralization requiring re-moralization (Frank, 2002). My 'dependence'-inducing practice could have been re-authored as functional dependability leading to engagement toward a safe container for healing from injustice and abuse.

In this way I am re-authoring my own personal narrative in ways that encompass the personal and professional growth I experience through my work with trauma survivors. The journey 'back from the edge' was a defining moment in my development as a psychotherapist and remains a work in progress.

---

### Reflective exercise

One way of beginning to reflect and write your own practice narratives is to keep a journal. Here are a few simple hints to getting started in writing about your own practice and how it can reveal themes in your life story.

Begin with a simple meditation or period of silence to quiet and focus the mind. Find a regular time and place in your home where you can be alone with the thoughts of the day. Often first thing in the morning or last thing before you go to bed at night can be quiet times in many households.

Write whatever comes to your mind in the moment without judgement or censure. It might be something you found funny or sad at work, something that is worrying you, or people around you at home or work about whom you are dealing with more negative feelings. It might be a feeling of gratitude to a person or for something that has happened.

To begin with you might focus your thinking by choosing a critical incident in your practice or professional life, that is, *an incident that in your view was the one from which you learned something vital*. Write down what happened factually from your own perspective, that is, write from the 'I'. It might be one incident or a series of events that are related in some way. For example, you might choose a complex client you worked with over a number of years who posed many issues for you. You might write about an ethical and moral dilemma or an event that pushed your buttons or violated an important belief/value that you hold dear. Notice the tension if one exists in the scenario you choose to write about. It could be a success story about your work or an important relationship with a colleague in your workplace.

In writing be aware of the choices you make in how you word your experience, the language you use; which aspects you decide to include and emphasize. Be aware of any emotions you are experiencing as you re-visit this incident by writing. Try to note down the gaps, biases and themes that you notice (in the process of deconstructing the event by remembering it and writing about what happened).

- Who might be the potential people involved in the incident or affected by it (either directly or indirectly)?
- What is your position in relation to these people?
- What was your interpretation of the incident then?
- Whose perspectives are represented in writing this incident?
- What knowledge or theory has informed your interpretation? (This can be both formal and informal knowledge.)
- What assumptions and personal values informed your interpretation of the incident?
- Thinking about this incident today, what is your interpretation of the incident?
- What (if any) new learning have you gained/or not gained from it?
- How might you be better or worse as a result of the incident?
- Now that you have finished writing – how has the process of writing been for you?
- What emotions are evoked and where are you now having written this?
- Take a moment to reflect and write any comments about the process of writing your reflection on practice.

## References

Bacon, V. (2013). Yarning and listening. In B. Bennett, S. Green, S. Gilbert and D. Bessarab (Eds). (2013). *Our voices: Aboriginal and Torres Strait Islander social work* (pp. 136–165). South Yarra, Palgrave Macmillan.

Bates, G. (2006). On being a therapist: Perspectives and conversations – Roundtable discussion. Australian Family Therapy Conference and the Gestalt Australia and New Zealand (GANZ) Conference, Hilton on the Park, Melbourne, Australia.

Bonnano, G. (2004). Loss, trauma and human resilience: Have we underestimated the human capacity to thrive after extremely aversive events? *American Psychologist, 59* (1), 20–8.

Briere, J. (1996). *Therapy for adults molested as children: Beyond survival* (2nd edn, revised and expanded). New York: Springer.

Coffey, R. (1998). *Unspeakable truths and happy endings: Human cruelty and the new trauma therapy.* New York: Sidran Press.

Collins, S. (2008a). Social workers, resilience, positive emotions and optimism. *Practice: Social Work in Action, 19* (4), 255–69.

Collins, S. (2008b). Statutory social workers, job satisfaction, coping, social support and individual differences. *British Journal of Social Work, 38* (6), 1173–93.

Collins, S. and Long, A. (2003). Working with the psychological effects of trauma: Consequences for mental health care workers – A literature review. *Journal of Psychiatric and Mental Health Nursing, 10*, 417–24.

Courtois, C. A. (1988). *Healing the incest wound: Adult survivors in therapy.* New York: W. W. Norton.

Courtois, C. A. (1997). Healing the incest wound: A treatment update with attention to recovered memory issues. *American Journal of Psychotherapy, 51* (4), 464–96.

Cunningham, M. (2003). Impact of trauma work on social work clinicians: Empirical findings. *Social Work, 48* (4), 451–9.

Dalenberg, C. (2000). *Countertransference and the treatment of trauma.* La Jolla, CA: American Psychological Association.

Figley, C. R. (Ed). (1995). *Compassion fatigue: Secondary traumatic stress disorder from treating the traumatised.* New York: Brunner/Mazel.

Figley, C. R. (Ed.). (2006). *Mapping trauma and its wake: Autobiographic essays by pioneer trauma scholars.* New York: Routledge.

Frank, A. W. (2002). Relations of caring: Demoralisation and remoralisation in the clinic. *International Journal for Human Caring, 6* (2), 13–19.

Grosch, W. N. and Olsen, D. C. (1994). *When helping starts to hurt: A new look at burnout among psychotherapists.* New York: Norton.

Harms, L. (2015). *Understanding trauma and resilience.* London: Palgrave Macmillan.

Hart, B. (1995). Re-authoring the stories we work by: Situating the narrative approach in the presence of the family of therapists. *Australian and New Zealand Journal of Family Therapy, 16* (4), 181–9.

Herman, J. (1992). *Trauma and recovery.* New York: Basic Books.

Jacobs, L. (2007). Pacific Gestalt Institute's winter retreat lecture [audiotape]. Santa Barbara, CA. Used with the permission of author.

Joyce, P. and Sills, C. (2001). *Skills in gestalt counselling and psychotherapy.* London: SAGE.

Kepner, J. I. (1987). *Body process: Working with the body in psychotherapy.* San Francisco, CA: Jossey-Bass.

Kepner, J. I. (2003a). The embodied field. *British Gestalt Journal, 12* (1), 6–14.

Kepner, J. I. (2003b). *Healing tasks: Psychotherapy with adult survivors of childhood abuse.* Cambridge, MA: Gestalt Institute Press.

MacKewn, J. (1997). *Developing gestalt counselling.* London: SAGE.

Myerhoff, B. (1982). *Number our days: Triumph of continuity and culture among Jewish old people in an urban ghetto.* New York: Simon and Schuster/Touchstone Books.

Myerhoff, B. (1992). *Remembered lives: The work of ritual, storytelling, and growing older.* Ann Arbor: University of Michigan Press.

Opie, A. (2000). *Thinking teams/thinking clients: Knowledge-based teamwork.* New York: Columbia University Press.

Pack, M. J. (2004). Sexual abuse counsellors' responses to stress and trauma: A social work perspective. *New Zealand Journal of Counselling, 25* (2), 1–17.

Pack, M. J. (2008). Back from the edge of the world: Re-authoring a story of practice using narrative and gestalt approaches. *Journal of Systemic Therapies, 27* (3), 25–39.

Pack, M. (2010). Career themes in the lives of sexual abuse counsellors. *New Zealand Journal of Counselling, 30* (2), 75–92.

Parlett, M. and Lee, R. G. (2005). Contemporary gestalt therapy: Field theory. In Woldt A. and Toman S. (Eds). *Gestalt therapy history: Theory and practice* (pp. 41–63). London: SAGE.

Parton, N. and O'Byrne, P. (2000). *Constructive social work.* Basingstoke: Macmillan.

Pearlman, L. A. and MacIan, P. S. (1995). Vicarious traumatisation: An empirical study of the effects of trauma work on trauma therapists. *Professional Psychology: Research and Practice, 26* (6), 558–65.

Pearlman, L. A. and Saakvitne, K. W. (1995). *Trauma and the therapist: Countertransference and vicarious traumatisation in psychotherapy with incest survivors.* New York: Norton.

Pearlman, L. A., Saakvitne, K. W. and staff of the Traumatic Stress Institute. (1996). *Transforming the pain: A workbook on vicarious traumatisation for helping professionals who work with traumatised clients.* New York: Norton.

Smith, L. T. (1999). *Decolonising methodologies: Research and Indigenous peoples.* Dunedin: Zed Books.

Trotter, C. (1999). *Working with involuntary clients.* London: SAGE.

White, M. (1995). *Re-authoring lives: Interviews and essays.* Adelaide: Dulwich Centre.

White, M. (1997). *Narratives of therapists' lives: Interviews and essays.* Adelaide: Dulwich Centre.

White, M. and Epston, D. (1990). *Narrative means to therapeutic ends.* Adelaide: Dulwich Centre.

Yalom, I. D. (1989). *Love's executioner and other tales of psychotherapy.* New York: Basic Books.

Zinker, J. (1977). *Creative process in gestalt psychotherapy.* New York: Vintage Books.

## Further reading

The following references provide foundational knowledge about narrative theory and healing from trauma from differing perspectives. Some are foundational theory-building (White and Epston, and Myerhoff), others look at narrative from a cultural (Bacon) perspective or wider systems perspectives (Harms):

Bacon, V. (2013). Yarning and listening. In Bennett B., Green S., Gilbert S. and Bessarab D. (Eds). (2013). *Our voices: Aboriginal and Torres Strait Islander social work.* South Yarra: Palgrave Macmillan.

Harms, L. (2015). *Understanding trauma and resilience.* London: Palgrave Macmillan.

Hart, B. (1995). Re-authoring the stories we work by: Situating the narrative approach in the presence of the family of therapists. *Australian and New Zealand Journal of Family Therapy*, *16* (4), 181–9.

Myerhoff, B. (1982). *Number our days: Triumph of continuity and culture among Jewish old people in an urban ghetto.* New York: Simon and Schuster/Touchstone Books.

Myerhoff, B. (1992). *Remembered lives: The work of ritual, storytelling, and growing older.* Ann Arbor: University of Michigan Press.

White, M. (1995). *Re-authoring lives: Interviews and essays.* Adelaide: Dulwich Centre.

White, M. (1997). *Narratives of therapists' lives: Interviews and essays.* Adelaide: Dulwich Centre.

White, M. and Epston, D. (1990). *Narrative means to therapeutic ends.* Adelaide: Dulwich Centre.

# Chapter 4

# Relationships and how vicarious traumatization can impact significant others

Steve: From a sexual point of view I hardly feel like being adventurous in case it crosses one of her boundaries and reminds her of the sexual abuse she has just been working with for the last month. So from that point of view our sexual intimacy has taken a dive and gone very quiet.

Tony: Certainly there is something that is the back of your mind that has to be dealt with. But in the back of my mind there is a view that says: 'I wouldn't dare be adventurous in any way'. I'm not like this, but imagine if you started to get out a whip and garters and things like that. God! For a person who is counselling sexual abuse people, you just wouldn't dare.

*Two husbands of the counsellor-participants discuss changes in their relationships*

## Introduction

Physical intimacy was an area that the husbands of the counsellor-participants discussed as being negatively impacted by their wives involvement in sexual abuse therapy as Steve and Tony explain in the above excerpts from their interviews for my research. Not surprisingly psychotherapists' effectiveness in working with survivors of trauma is dependent on the quality of personal and professional support they access and use (Pearlman and Saakvitne, 1995). Therefore, if there are problems with withdrawal and isolation in intimate relationships in the therapist's life, separation from a source of sustenance may become real, removing a potential buffer to vicarious traumatization. This chapter, drawing from the larger study reported in Chapters 2 and 3, focuses on the experience of the significant others of the trauma therapists interviewed (Pack, 2010). The literature on vicarious traumatization has suggested that the support of significant others, or conversely the lack of it, is a key variable in how effectively counsellors approach and deal with the rigours of trauma-related helping (Pearlman and Saakvitne, 1995). Using in-depth interviews and a qualitative research methodology, counsellor-participants were interviewed for the wider study to elicit their views of the framework and the impact of the work on intimacy and relationships. The focus of this chapter is on the subsequent interviews with the counsellor-participants' family (the personal significant others) and colleagues (professional significant others) to explore their awareness of alterations in the counsellor-participants' beliefs as experienced in their relationships with the counsellor-participants over time (Pack, 2010). The term 'dual significant' other is used to refer to a professional significant other of the counsellor-participant who later became a life partner or friend.

The findings of the study indicate that while the personal significant others did not use the same terminology as the professional significant others, their descriptions of changes they experienced in relation to the counsellor-participants mirrored the literature. Those personal significant others who were outside the trauma-counselling discourse drew upon frameworks of knowledge that were quite different from, and in some instances in conflict with, the paradigms used by the counsellor-participants. They reported that their relationships with the counsellor-participants were transformed over time as different personal priorities and values from their own were identified (Pack, 2010).

## Background

As discussed in Chapter 1, workers employed in a variety of front-line positions engage with survivors of trauma on a daily basis. The effects of this work can include an erosion of trust and esteem of others, and disruptions to the worker's sense of the world as a safe place (Cunningham, 2003). These shifts in belief and world view have been connected to the experience of working intensively with trauma disclosures and more specifically with work involving interpersonal violence (Moulden and Firestone, 2007). As discussed in Chapter 2, vicarious traumatization is a process that occurs when psychotherapists' sense of self and world view are negatively transformed through empathetic engagement with traumatic disclosures from clients (Pearlman and Saakvitne, 1995). The effects are considered to be cumulative, permanent and irreversible (Pearlman and Saakvitne, 1995). Traditionally vicarious traumatization has been studied and researched from the perspective of clinical psychology, as the original research on vicarious traumatization was undertaken with and by clinical psychologists who were working with sexual abuse survivors. This framework along with allied concepts of burnout and compassion fatigue is now being applied to other trauma workers' experiences such as social workers (Clemans, 2004; Cranfield, 2005; Cunningham, 2003), psychotherapists (Moulden and Firestone, 2007), telephone helpline counsellors (Dunkley and Whelan, 2006b), police and paramedics (Figley, 1995; Follette *et al.*, 1994), mental health professionals (Collins and Long, 2003; Sabin-Farrell and Turpin, 2003) and nurses (Sabo, 2006).

In particular, the relational distancing from others, cynicism and detachment experienced by trauma workers as a process associated with vicarious traumatization has continued to be discussed in the research literature (Collins and Long, 2003; Cunningham, 2003; Dunkley and Wheelan, 2006a, 2006b). Difficulty in modulating emotions and relationship difficulties are 'potentially the result of emotional withdrawal which can be the result of vicarious traumatization' (Wastell, 2005: 124). Johnson (1993) recommended that future research on social workers working with survivors of domestic abuse focus on the impact of the work on their relationships to more fully explore this process. However, the views of family, friends and colleagues remain largely undocumented in the literature on vicarious traumatization to the present day.

The support of professional peers and what I have termed the 'professional significant others' is central to trauma therapists' continued wellness and effectiveness on the job. Fox and Cooper (1998) use the conceptual framework of vicarious traumatization to investigate the effects of client suicide on psychotherapists in private practice. Drawing on two extended case vignettes they conclude that the support of colleagues is pivotal to enabling trauma workers to cope with suicidal clients. They recommend that those working with suicidal clients form group practices for education, support and sharing. These informal and formal networks assist in ensuring accountability and a working through of often painful feelings that arise for the worker (Fox and Cooper, 1998: 155–6).

## Research aims

Following the larger research study of the counsellor-participants reported in Chapter 2, I now move to focus on the second phase of the research with the significant others of the therapists (Pack, 2008). The purpose of this chapter, therefore, is to focus on the impacts of work in the field of trauma on the families and colleagues of the counsellor- participants earlier discussed. My training and experience as a social worker had raised my awareness of the importance of searching for alternative sources of knowledge that had not been heard before, or fell outside the dominant discourse on vicarious traumatization. These sources of knowledge, though unavailable often as published sources, flourish as stories recounted informally in work and private domains. Thus, I became interested in the narratives of the counsellors' significant others and wished to explore their narratives as 'subjugated knowledge', referred to in passing within the wider vicarious traumatization literature (Pack, 2008).

The intention of the interviews with the significant others nominated by the counsellor-participants was to assemble three perspectives on the theme of the effects of vicarious traumatization. The counsellor-participants' responses were supplemented by the viewpoints of two sets of 'significant others': those colleagues working in the same field as the therapist (professional significant others) and personal friends and family (personal significant others). I compare and contrast the three perspectives in terms of the issues they raised during individual, in-depth, semi-structured interviews with the three groups: the counsellor-participants, their family and friends, and professional significant others. The topics they discussed included the effects of the work on the therapist in ways that are congruent with McCann and Pearlman's (1990) framework surrounding the cognitive shifts that occur in safety, trust, dependency, intimacy and esteem of others. However, several major themes were identified from the interviews that went beyond the conceptual framework of vicarious traumatization, which were highlighted by the qualitative research design and methodology (Pack, 2010).

## Methodology

I aimed to explore three viewpoints on a theme by researching the 'triads' of the counsellor-participants and their nominated personal and professional significant others. Similarities and differences could then be noted within the triads and across the groupings and analysed using 'pattern-matching' (Yin, 1985) in which each triad was analysed for internal consistency and the same frame used to analyse the themes across the triads.

Using a semi-structured interview schedule, nominated significant others were asked to comment on their perceptions of the counsellor-participant over the period in which they had known them. Did they consider the work had impacted on the counsellor-participant in any way over time? Different accounts of the history of their relationship, its ups and downs, were woven into the discussion. Then I explored how the significant others accounted for the themes and patterns discussed in relation to the counsellor-participant and the relationship of which they were a part. I defined another group of significant others who had begun as colleagues and moved into personal friendships and intimate relationships. I asked the personal or 'dual' significant others if they considered there had been any effects for them of living with a counsellor doing trauma therapy. I found it was this question, answered from their own perspectives, that sparked their interest in the topic, so this is where I decided to begin the interview (Pack, 2008).

## Selection of 'significant others'

I asked the counsellor-participants to nominate a personal and professional significant other to be interviewed. Initially I had assumed that counsellor-participants would want to nominate two different individuals who represented the dimensions of support offered by a colleague or work associate (professional significant other), and those dimensions offered by a spouse, friend or family member (personal significant other). In practice, I discovered that these distinctions between the personal and the professional did not readily fit the experience of many of the counsellor-participants.

## Ethical issues

As with the larger study of the counsellor-participants reported in Chapter 2, ethical approval was obtained prior to the commencement of the fieldwork. In agreeing to the interview I requested that participants signed a consent form to enable the material to be transcribed and used in an unidentified form using pseudonyms of their choosing. I made every effort to write in such a way as to avoid including any information that might identify any individual. In some cases I chose to cluster responses and summarize themes due to the sensitive nature of the material and to avoid any unintentional breach of confidentiality through direct use of quotations from participants.

Each participant was asked to identify a support person to be available should the interview raise personal issues that needed to be further discussed. At the completion of each interview I checked as to the availability of a support person to deal with any feelings raised during the interview and to debrief. All participants were asked to indicate whether they wished the recording of their interview to be returned and whether they wished to be sent a copy of the final summary of the research. Three participants wished for their own interview transcripts to be returned to them on completion of the research as they found their contributions illuminating of key personal issues they wished to further reflect upon.

All but one of the interviews were conducted on an individual basis to preserve individual confidentiality. The exception to this was two adult children who wished to be interviewed together about their parent. I advised participants that any material raised in one interview would not be disclosed in any other interview.

## Characteristics of significant others

The division between the personal and the professional blurred, as the counsellors had spent many years in this area of clinical practice and had gravitated socially towards colleagues who were like-minded in their personal philosophies who became life friends and partners.

Table 4.1 summarizes the key characteristics of those significant others.

## Themes from the interviews

As I commenced interviewing, I realized that my assumption that significant others were 'supporters' of the counsellors was incorrect. There were some personal significant others who seemed to resent the personal growth that went with the counsellors' experiences of counselling in the trauma field. I often heard from personal significant others that they felt left behind or relegated to the role of being the practical, behind-the-scenes person. Professional significant others, too, were sometimes critical of the foibles and habits of their colleague, relating to me in psychological terminology the reasons for their criticisms.

**TABLE 4.1** Characteristics of the significant others of the counsellor-participants

| | Age range (years) | Self-identified as (careers) | Length of relationship with counsellor-participant | Ethnicity and gender – self-identified | Relationship to counsellor-participant |
|---|---|---|---|---|---|
| Personal significant other | 18–59 | Student<br>Unemployed<br>Retired<br>Builder<br>Nun<br>Spiritual director<br>Insurance manager<br>Rehabilitation worker | 17–33 years | Māori* (1)<br>Samoan/Pākehā** (2)<br>Pākehā (9)<br><br>Male (9)<br>Female (3) | Adult children<br>Friends<br>Husbands<br>Partners |
| Professional significant other | 38–60 | Counsellor<br>Clinical psychologist<br>Psychotherapist<br>Social worker<br>Clinical supervisor | 5–15 years | Māori (1)<br>Pākehā (4)<br><br>Female (4)<br>Male (1) | Colleagues<br>Clinical supervisors<br>Work associates<br>Professional peers/advisors |
| Dual role significant other (professional significant others who became life partners) | 46–60 | as above | 5–11 years | Pākehā (5)<br><br>Female (5) | Business partners<br>Employees<br>Work colleagues<br>Clinical supervisors<br>Teachers who later became friends and life partners with the counsellor-participants |

* Māori is a term that refers to a New Zealander who is indigenous to New Zealand
** Pākehā is a term that refers to a New Zealander of European descent

Adapted from Pack (2010)

Personal significant others did not have this shared frame of reference and, hence, did not easily recognize the forces behind the personal transformation that they observed in the counsellor. I discovered in talking with the counsellor-participants and their nominated personal significant others that misunderstandings and miscommunications were more likely to arise in their relationships, in the absence of this shared frame of reference. These miscommunications were instances of 'talking past each other' in a cultural sense (Metge and Kinloch, 1978). This 'talking past each other' had implications for the quality and longevity of the counsellor–personal significant other relationships. This concept involved two sub-themes. The first of these themes involved the counsellors feeling met or matched emotionally by their professional significant others attuning accurately to their needs. Second, that professional or dual role significant others affirmed and understood the search for meaning and experiences that was evoked by the counsellor-participants' work, and their own histories, which the personal significant others could not. Like individuals belonging to different ethnic tribes or cultures who speak different languages, there were miscommunications based in a gulf of understanding between the lived experiences of the counsellor-participants and significant others who did not share their experience of their work with sexual abuse disclosures. I have conceptualized this 'talking past each other' as occurring within the relationships of the counsellor-participants to their husbands, friends and children (Pack, 2010). These themes are discussed in relation to the psychological needs identified in the original self-constructivist theory: intimacy, safety, trust and esteem (Pearlman and Saakvitne, 1995). These core needs will be explored with the three groups of significant others: the personal partners, husbands, friends and family; the professional significant others – colleagues, peers and supervisors; and the dual professional others who began as professional associates but moved into becoming friends and in some cases partners, while retaining alliances across the therapy work lines (Pack, 2010).

First we turn to the partners and husbands of the counsellor-participants to explore what the impact had been on these areas of their relating.

## Intimacy and relationships

Husbands saw an increasing intolerance with the behaviour of men as being more directly connected with their wives' work in the sexual abuse field. These were husbands who interpreted the comments from the counsellor-participants about men in general, as applying to them more personally. For one marriage, the expectations of the counsellor-participant made it difficult for her husband, Steve, to behave as he usually did without feeling judged and labelled as being 'chauvinistic' and 'aggressive' or 'depressed', he told me. This made everyday life more complicated and difficult to navigate his way through. He conceptualized some of the changes he observed as being related to her work as a trauma therapist:

> Steve: Her tolerance level about any abuse of any sort has diminished. I think she would be very vocal if anything cropped up in the family about those kinds of issues. As I've said, I've just been thinking about this aspect. About the time that she was learning about violence and going through these changes, I got labelled as being violent and I reacted quite strongly against that … I think, over time, she has realized that it's not necessarily violence and it's certainly not aimed at her. So her attitudes have modified a little bit. I don't know quite what she thinks about me now. But I wouldn't be surprised if she put that label on me over those issues.

These attitudes had implications for the husbands' sense of closeness and intimacy within the relationship. The space to be oneself and to express oneself was missing. Friends were selected who would understand his point of view, so that one of the husbands interviewed went to live in another city and found emotional closeness in a relationship outside the marriage.

The husbands who were married to the counsellor-participants interviewed told me that they were increasingly mindful of being a man, and the power attached to men's significance in society. For some this led to a tendency to retreat into the sidelines of gender debates to avoid these dilemmas as far as possible. For other husbands, the challenges inherent in their masculinity led them to join men's groups to educate other men about male sexuality and the power and control issues that stemmed from being a man in New Zealand society.

Physical intimacy was often discussed by husbands as problematic with wives who were working as trauma therapists with sexual abuse survivors. This was seen within the context of the nature of the work by husbands and the emotional detachment that they saw resulting from work-related demands. However, husbands' sensitivity to being perceived by their counsellor wives as less than politically correct in dealings with women seemed also to alter the dynamics of the relationship. One of the counsellors' husbands explained to me that he considered his wife's expectations of him had changed in the area of physical intimacy. He said he struggled to know what was 'appropriate' conduct for him in that aspect of their relationship and had 'given up trying'.

Three long-term committed relationships of counsellors had ended over the duration of the study. These separations seemed prompted by the desire for a different kind of relationship based in a greater understanding of the work of the counsellor-participant and their growth as individuals. The counsellor-participants considered this personal evolution had been brought about by their empathetic engagement with clients who had been sexually abused. This engagement was reported to have changed many aspects of their lives, including their personal relationships.

## Friendships

Significant others who were women described greater cynicism about men in general and identified more closely with the survivor of abuse. This view mirrors Johnson's (1993) and Johnson and Hunter's (1997) findings and connects with the literature surrounding previous trauma history of sexual abuse therapists and links to the potential for vicarious traumatization (Folette et al., 1994; Pearlman and MacIan, 1995; Sabin-Farrell and Turpin, 2003). The counsellor-participants often guessed when women friends had been abused and made suggestions as to where to seek help. For Natalie, a dual significant other (i.e. a colleague and a friend), the assistance of Hayley, one of the counsellor-participants, helped her in dealing with her early childhood abuse. Both women were able to relate to one another the circumstances of their own abuse. This sharing of experience about many areas of their lives, including their traumatic pasts, provided a shared frame of reference. Their differing responses to expressing their own anger was discussed as an early challenge within their relationship. In the face of trauma disclosures, however, these 'personality differences' were set aside in the interests of working together.

For Mary and Rose, this shared frame of reference developed over a decade where each increasingly valued the relationship of the other despite differences of style and personality. In the following passage, Mary remembers her early impressions of her work colleague, Rose. Both were social workers in their early training with Mary working as a family therapist and Rose as a community worker. Both then retrained as psychotherapists working with sexual abuse survivors. Mary noticed that her respect and esteem of Rose had deepened with Rose's continued personal growth over the years, arising from their participation in personal therapy. Mary increasingly valued her friendship with Rose as a consequence of recognizing their respective personal journeys which had brought them to setting up as a group counselling practice:

> Mary: I found it [Rose's anger] quite hard to cope with actually. I found it quite hard dealing with other people's anger too. I think as we have both continued our personal development work and become more comfortable with a range of our own feelings that's changed. I was also very aware of her coming from quite a different work background. I had no idea what that meant, I couldn't make sense of it [laughs]. And now Rose and some of my closest friends are working or have worked in that field.

## Parenting and safety

The literature on vicarious traumatization and secondary traumatization had suggested that counsellors' beliefs about their own personal safety and that of their loved ones were affected by the work, as a normal response to contact with traumatic material (Figley, 1995; McCann and Pearlman, 1990; Pearlman and Saakvitne, 1995). Adult daughters talked about the protectiveness of their counsellor-participant mothers at the time when they were rebelling against parental restrictions. Later they appreciated the limits provided. This period of rebellion had unfortunate consequences in that the more protective the counsellor-participant mothers became, the more their daughters told me they had engaged in risk-taking behaviour with friends. Sometimes, this resulted in these teenagers having some experience themselves of abuse. Hana, an adult daughter of one of the counsellor-participants, talked of an incident in which she had put herself in a situation of danger when she had been rebelling against her mother's wishes as a teenager. The separation of her parents also coloured her experience of home at that time:

> Hana: Well, things like when I was younger, and I first started wanting to go out, she was a lot more careful than a lot of parents. Because she knows, what happens. Yeah, and if I did [go out], she wanted to know where I was going and who was going to be there and stuff. Well, it used to make me quite mad because my other friends could go out and also because my Dad let me go out. So, I used to have big fights with her about it. For about a year we were always fighting, but you know, I stopped and now we're friends.

For adult children of the counsellor-participants, they described being responsible at a young age due to their awareness of parental emotional detachment and/or unavailability. Hana thought that she had taken on more parental responsibility as a consequence of her mother's work: 'Well, I was only quite young when she started [counselling], but I think I then started worrying. I am more worried than I would be if she didn't do the work. And I think I'm also more responsible.'

A theme among the adult children was that they wished that their parents, who worked as psychotherapists, would be like their friends' parents and avoid counselling them at home. Hana's mother and father were both counsellors. Like Jesse and Sam, two daughters of another counsellor-participant, Hana was appreciative of the sensitivity with which her parents tried to understand her feelings. However, sometimes, she said she disliked being 'therapized':

> Hana: I should have said this earlier. She used, I don't think she does it consciously, but she'd, like, counsel me. [Sigh] … Well, um, the things that they say, like you can tell a counsellor's statements from a non-counsellor, because they'll say things like: 'Why don't you tell me how you feel about that.' Oh, I don't know, things like that. I think you come to recognize it after a while. Oh, they'd say, like with my Dad, I'd be like really, really angry with him, and he'd be like: 'Are you sure you're angry with me?' And I'd be like: 'Yes!' [Gasp of exasperation].

## Balancing work, play and family life

For personal significant others, who lacked the theoretical knowledge about the impact of work in the trauma therapy area, the changes observed in the counsellor-participant were less easy to understand. There was a sense in which personal significant others found the counsellor-participants emotionally absent, though physically present, at the end of the working day. Concerns about the tiredness of counsellor-participants, which was sometimes linked to sleep difficulties, emotional fatigue and overwork, was a major worry expressed. Sam and Jesse discussed their mother's sleep problems since beginning to work in the sexual abuse field. Her tiredness meant that they thought she feigned listening to their news at the end of the day. They were aware that she was too fatigued to absorb any more and so walked away:

> I sometimes get annoyed by how tired she is, and I think anyone's life has so much stuff in it and imagine dealing with all these other people's. And I just sometimes think she loves it [being a counsellor] above anything else and that's awesome. And I think that's excellent and love her for doing that, but, at the same time, I don't know how I could do it. So it takes so much energy from so many places that I sometimes wish she would look after herself a bit more, like, rest. She's a bit of a workaholic.

Geoff, husband to Jill, one of the counsellor-participants, hoped she would decide to pursue her creative writing and artistic pursuits from home, in addition to, or instead of, working as a trauma therapist with sexual abuse survivors. Her work as a trauma therapist was seen as taking her away from the family both physically and emotionally, from his perspective. He talked longingly of the time when the family would not rely on her income from her private practice as a therapist, so that she had the choice of taking on fewer cases, or, in time, leaving the therapy field. He reflected on his own responses to his partner's work as a therapist:

> Geoff: I suppose, really, in some ways I get resentful about it [Jill's involvement in counselling] and I suppose if I think about over those 14 years, I think it's bad to be resentful because here are people who have huge traumas in their life. And I think sometimes I'm resentful about the space it's taken, which is why I like Jill being either a teacher and doing some supervision or a small amount of counselling. I never thought that I was resentful but I think I have been at times.

For the dual significant others who were partners to the counsellor-participant and themselves working as trauma therapists, there was a level of support available that was not usually a feature of the personal significant other–counsellor-participant relationships. Thus, one partner talked about some evenings turning into 'an extended supervision session' that dealt with the counsellor-participant's issues and responses to particular cases that were complex in some way, or where the client remained at risk. However, there was also aware-ness that these sessions caused strain to their relationship, as her dual significant other said she did not like talking about casework at home yet the informal debriefing continued.

## Debriefing, support, supervision and parallel processes

Professional and dual significant others recognized that vicarious traumatization was a fact of life that needed to be worked with using a variety of strategies. Often in talking about themes in their relationships, professional and dual significant others made connec-tions between the parallel processes they were unconsciously engaged in that were linked to the traumatic disclosures from clients and the dynamics of the therapeutic relationship. Transference and countertransference coloured the relationships among colleagues within the organization due to the nature of their work with trauma.

A poignant example was from a dual role significant other, Douglas, who found that, on reflection, he became dissociated in observing and assisting his colleague to deal with his dissociative states following contact with traumatized clients. Dissociation, common to the experience of many trauma survivors, is conceptualized by Kepner (2003) as being a normal response in which the body may go on acting as it does but inwardly the body is felt to be acting in a dream-like reality, and has a contagion-like effect on others. This is a common countertransferential response when working with sexual abuse survivors who are them-selves dissociated. Kepner describes the psychic withdrawal out of the body into dissociative states of consciousness as having a protective function for the survivor but if unattended has the effect of compromising the self-awareness of the counsellor. Sometimes the self and the body are experienced as disembodied in a persistent way, for others it is more temporary and fleeting. Inevitably this impacted the counsellor-participant's relationships. For the male therapists, they described a range of obstacles to relationships with women.

> Douglas: One of the things that has affected my personal relationships, yes it has, I'm in no doubt at all about that, it has made it a lot more difficult to relate to women because one of the things is, I'm almost unconsciously looking for trauma. And then I with-draw, so that's an issue. And yet some of my closest friends are women who've been traumatized, so, I mean, that ends up being simply a friendship though, because there is probably some work I need to do in that area myself.

The witnessing of accounts of trauma by the counsellor-participants and their professional others came at a cost to their relationships if the underlying dynamics were unrecognized. Learning to balance the client's own hope and despair with one's own was considered crucial to maintaining therapeutic effectiveness. As one of the counsellor-participants reminds us:

> Sally: What we are about with clients is about how to help them in transforming their lives from seeing all of the 90 per cent of their lives as the problem to seeing the 10 per cent of the hope and the solution.

## A pause to reflect

As therapists working in the field of trauma it is important to ask those around you whom you share your life with if vicarious traumatization is affecting your relationships with them. The literature suggests that those closest to the therapist often observe subtle and not so subtle effects as we have seen in the significant others' comments in this chapter. It is important to ask if any of these themes have relevance from their experiences. For example, the following questions might be helpful to ask your professional and personal supporters:

- Have you ever felt upset or threatened in any way by the work that I do with trauma survivors?
- Do you like me doing this work? Why?
- What have you noticed about me and my responses to you over the time I have been engaged as a trauma therapist?
- Has my response/attitude to you changed in any way over time? How?
- Can you give me an example of this?

As a therapist you also need to take stock of the impact of the work on your relationships periodically by self-reflection. The following questions focus thinking about changes in your relationships.

What changes do you see in your relationships within your social networks, including:

1. Partners, husbands, wives and lovers?
2. Friends, family members and children?
3. Neighbours, acquaintances and work colleagues?
4. Strangers?
5. Are your professional networks becoming your personal networks?
6. What mix of personal and professional relationships do you wish to have in your life?
7. Do you have the right balance of the personal and the professional in your relationships?
8. Where do you need to make changes?

## Conclusion

Further research is needed to explore the effects of the counsellor-participants' professional networks becoming also their personal networks, over time. For the personal significant others of counsellors, education about the transformation they are likely to encounter in relation to their spouse, partner or parent may enable a greater awareness and appreciation of vicarious traumatization and a working-through of the issues of intimacy and trust. Just as therapists have responsibility to self-monitor and develop their own self-care programmes, significant others have a vested interest in ensuring this occurs in practice and can be co-supporters of this process. If family and friends, clinical supervisors and colleagues are aware of the signs and symptoms, they can reflect to the therapist when and how vicarious traumatization seems to be impacting and assist them to address the issue.

Within the specialized training about vicarious traumatization, the personal significant others of helping professionals require a parallel education and support network to be effective allies in the therapist's ongoing programme of self-assessment and self-care. Topics to be addressed in such training could include 'the awareness, balance, connection model' developed by Pearlman *et al.* (1996). Second, involvement in 'meaning-making' activities such as reviewing individual and family goals and interests on a regular basis, spirituality, celebration, and social and community connection are important to integrate into one's lifestyle. Fostering humour, inner peace and a sense of connection with others together with an attitude of 'optimistic perseverance' are recommended (Medeiros and Prochaska, 1988). Creating a climate in which communication about the effects of vicarious traumatization can be openly discussed together with an exploration of how vicarious traumatization may be impacting on the individual is essential to maintaining effective practice as a therapist as well as an emotionally present and responsive partner, friend and parent.

A central dilemma of this research is how to approach and write about the participants' experience richly to retain the individual voices alongside the central themes identified, while avoiding the identification of individuals. The participants told me that they wished for me to share their narratives in the hope that it would illuminate a 'common' experience for others to learn from. The involvement of the focus group engaged in ongoing reflection provided feedback at each stage of the research was one way of accomplishing this aim. The discussions I initiated among the focus group members became constitutive of the research into vicarious traumatization through their critical-reflective process. Through discussing their own experiences of vicarious traumatization and practice dilemmas, their combined practice wisdom enabled me to formulate practical insights into vicarious traumatization that I used to formulate my own original theories. However, I was aware of the hazards of generalizing when, as Geertz (1988) suggests, researchers are engaged in writing 'fictions' that are composed of interpretations of interpretations. New literary styles are needed to research and write about qualitative research on such sensitive topics with under-researched groups that ensure confidentiality yet allow for the narratives of each participant to be heard.

## Bringing the narratives together: Mark's story – learning to 'play a low profile'

Some partners and husbands found creative ways to be supportive to their partners' and wives' counselling work over time. Important in this role was their ability, as they saw it, to absent oneself and to 'play a low profile'. Some felt uneasy when their partners or wives were seeing clients for therapy from their home private practice. Gardens, garden sheds and outdoor work offered a sanctuary to retreat to when clients were seen at home. These were seen as 'safe places' free from possible intrusion, from being around areas where they could overhear what was being said. Mark, married to Sally, one of the counsellor-participants, had found over their 30-year marriage how to support his wife and maintain privacy for the client simultaneously in the following excerpt from his interview. He worked as an insurance manager but when he was at home and his wife was seeing clients in the home where she had her private counselling room, he chose to seek such a sanctuary:

Mark: It's not a problem [therapy happening at home]. Most of it is done when I'm not around anyway and she has some sessions at the weekend. But it's not a small property so there are other places where you are out of earshot. I can find something to do that is half a mile away. I am working on the basis that clients would value privacy and confidentiality. The thought that they [trauma survivor clients] are being gawped at by some other clown – for heaven's sake – after what they have been through, they don't need that!

Unofficial helping was often part of the significant others' role, accepted philosophically as being part of the relationship. Ben, another partner of one of the counsellor-participants, was relieved he did not have to know very much about what his partner did while he was providing administrative support for her practice by running a few reports through the photocopier without looking at the text of what the report said.

Steve found that he did not confide in his wife as he felt analysed by her for political correctness towards his attitudes about women and domestic violence. He described being increasingly excluded from her support network so felt increasingly 'redundant':

Steve: I'm a good support when she has got, well, she did have a friend of ours dying; and when our kids are needing support. I'm good from that point of view and act as a normal husband in that role. But when it comes to support on an emotional need as a result of her job, or a business need as a result of her job, it goes entirely to someone else. Either to her supervisor or other close female friends, and they are, in fact, all female friends that she gets that kind of support from.

In the next chapters (5, 6 and 7) we explore some of the other support structures promoting trauma therapists' self-care involving clinical supervision, peer relationships/teamwork and the requirements of a comprehensive CISM programme in the organizational context.

# References

Clemans, S. E. (2004). Understanding vicarious traumatization: Strategies for social workers. *Social Work Today*, *4* (2), 13. Retrieved from www.socialworktoday.com/archive/swt_0204p13.htm (accessed 28 March 2008).

Cranfield, J. (2005). Secondary traumatisation, burnout, and vicarious traumatisation: A review of the literature as it relates to therapists who treat trauma. *Smith College Studies in Social Work*, *75* (2), 81–102.

Collins, S. and Long, A. (2003). Working with the psychological effects of trauma: Consequences for mental health care workers: A literature review. *Journal of Psychiatric and Mental Health Nursing*, *10* (4), 417–24.

Cunningham, M. (2003). Impact of trauma work on social work clinicians: Empirical findings. *Social Work*, *48* (4), 451–9.

Dunkley, J. and Whelan, T. A. (2006a). Vicarious traumatisation: Current status and future trends. *British Journal of Guidance and Counselling*, *34* (1), 107–17.

Dunkley, J. and Whelan, T. A. (2006b). Vicarious traumatisation in telephone counsellors: Internal and external influences. *British Journal of Guidance and Counselling*, *34* (4), 451–69.

Figley, C. R. (Ed.). (1995). *Compassion fatigue: Coping with secondary traumatic stress disorder in those who treat the traumatized.* New York: Brunner/Mazel.

Follette, V. M., Polusny, M. and Milbeck, K. (1994). Mental health and law enforcement professionals: Trauma history, psychological symptoms, and the impact of providing services to child sexual abuse survivors. *Professional Psychology: Research and Practice*, *25* (3), 275–82.

Fox, R. and Cooper, M. (1998). The effects of suicide on the private practitioner: A professional and personal perspective. *Clinical Social Work Journal*, *26* (2), 143–157.

Geertz, C. (1988). *Works and lives: The anthropologist as author.* Cambridge: Polity Press.

Johnson, C. (1993). Vicarious traumatisation: The experiences of counsellors working with sexual assault victims. An exploratory study. (Unpublished MA thesis). University of Newcastle, Sydney, Australia.

Johnson, C. N. E. and Hunter, M. (1997). Vicarious traumatisation in counsellors working in the New South Wales Assault Service: An exploratory study. *Work and Stress, 11* (4), 319–28.

Kepner, J. I. (2003). *Healing tasks: Psychotherapy with adult survivors of childhood abuse.* Cambridge, MA: Gestalt Institute Press.

McCann, I. L. and Pearlman, L. A. (1990). Vicarious traumatisation: A framework for understanding the psychological effects of working with victims. *Journal of Traumatic Stress, 3* (1), 131–49.

Medeiros, M. E. and Prochaska, J. O. (1988). Coping strategies that psychotherapists use in working with stressful clients. *Professional Psychology: Research and Practice, 19* (1), 112–14.

Metge, J. and Kinloch, P. (1978). *Talking past each other: Problems of cross-cultural communication.* Wellington: Victoria University Press.

Moulden, H. M. and Firestone, P. (2007). Vicarious traumatization: The impact on therapists who work with sexual offenders. *Trauma, Violence and Abuse, 8* (1), 67–83.

Pack, M. (2008). 'Back from the edge of the world': Re-authoring a story of practice with stress and trauma using Gestalt theories and narrative approaches. *Journal of Systemic Therapies, 27*(3), 30–44. doi: 10.1521/jsyt.2008.27.3.30, ISSN: 1195-4396

Pack, M. (2010). Transformation in progress: The effects of trauma on the significant others of sexual abuse therapists. *Qualitative Social Work Research and Practice, 9* (2), 249–65. doi: 10.1177/147332500936100

Pearlman, L. A. and MacIan, P. S. (1995). Vicarious traumatization: An empirical study of the effects of trauma work on trauma therapists. *Professional Psychology: Research and Practice, 26* (6), 558–65.

Pearlman, L. A. and Saakvitne, K. W. (1995). *Trauma and the therapist: Countertransference and in psychotherapy with incest survivors.* New York: Norton.

Pearlman, L. A., Saakvitne, K. W. and staff of the Traumatic Stress Institute. (1996). *Transforming the pain: A workbook on for helping professionals who work with traumatised clients.* New York: Norton.

Sabin-Farrell, R. and Turpin, G. (2003). Vicarious traumatization: Implications for the mental health of health workers? *Clinical Psychology Review, 23* (3), 449–80.

Sabo, B. M. (2006). Compassion fatigue and nursing work: Can we accurately capture the consequences of caring work? *International Journal of Nursing Practice, 12* (3), 136–42.

Wastell, C. (2005). *Understanding trauma and emotion: Dealing with trauma using an emotion-focused approach.* Maidenhead: Open University Press.

Yin, R. (1985). *Case study research.* New York: SAGE.

## Further reading

Dutton, M. A. (1992). *Empowering and healing the battered woman: A model for assessment and intervention.* New York: Springer.

Fook, J. (1993). *Radical casework: A theory of practice.* St Leonards, Australia: Allen & Unwin.

Fook, J. (Ed.). (1996). *The reflective researcher: Social workers' theories of practice Research.* St Leonards, Australia: Allen & Unwin.

Fook, J. (2002). *Social work: Critical theory and practice.* London: SAGE.

Fook, J. and Gardner, F. (Eds). (2007). *Practising critical reflection: A resource handbook.* Maidenhead: Open University Press.

Fook, J. and Pease, B. (Eds). (1999). *Transforming social work practice: Postmodern critical perspectives.* St Leonards, Australia: Allen & Unwin.

Fook, J., Ryan, M. and Hawkins, L. (2000). *Professional expertise: Practice, theory and education for working in uncertainty.* London: Whiting & Birch.

Fook, J., White, S. and Gardner, F. (Eds). (2006). *Critical reflection in health and social care.* St Leonards, Australia: Allen & Unwin.

Grosch, W. N. and Olsen, D. C. (1994). *When helping starts to hurt: A new look a burnout among psychotherapists.* New York: Norton.

Neumann, D. A. and Gamble, S. J. (1995). Issues in the professional development of psychotherapists: Countertransference and vicarious traumatization in the new therapist. *Psychotherapy, 32* (2), 341–7.

Rasmussen, B. (2005). An intersubjective perspective on vicarious trauma and its impact on the clinical process. *Journal of Social Work Practice, 19* (1), 19–30.

Sexton, L. (1999). Vicarious traumatization of counsellors and effects on their workplaces. *British Journal of Guidance and Counselling, 27* (3), 393–404.

Stamm, B. H. (Ed.) (1996). *Secondary traumatic stress: Self-care issues for clinicians, researchers and educators.* Lutherville, MD: Sidran Press.

Steed, L. G. and Downing, R. (1998). A phenomenological study of vicarious traumatisation among psychologists and professional counsellors working in the field of sexual abuse/assault. *Australasian Journal of Disaster and Trauma Studies, 2* (2), 1–8.

Stephens, C. (1997). Debriefing, social support and PTSD in the New Zealand police: Testing a multidimensional model of organisational traumatic stress. *Australasian Journal of Disaster and Trauma Studies, 1* (1), 321–40.

Stephens, C. and Long, N. (1997). The impact of trauma and social support on posttraumatic stress disorder: A study of New Zealand police officers. *Journal of Criminal Justice, 25* (4), 303–14.

# Chapter 5

# **Clinical supervision for trauma therapists**

## A liminal and dialogic space for reflection and self-care

### **Introduction**

I recognize that, that working in this field has also been very costly. The benefit for me, the richness, has been attending to my own and discovering my own inner resources. I guess you could call this inner growth 'spirituality'. I think this work [therapy] has certainly made it possible for me to focus and have much more awareness of my own need for growth.

*Ellen, consultant therapist discussing how the therapeutic relationship as a living process involved growth for the therapist and client. This interactive process and co-created space involved the dynamic and synergistic input of a clinical supervisor*

This chapter explores the needs of trauma therapists in clinical supervision and the models congruent with these needs. Drawing upon a systematic review of the literature on clinical supervision and subsequent research (Pack, 2009a, 2009b, 2015) building on my theorizing from earlier research (Pack, 2004), a relational approach to clinical supervision is recommended when dealing with trauma survivors as a therapist. Based in the underlying power dynamics in clinical supervision, themes in the relationship between the supervisor and supervisee and the challenges these pose for establishing clinical supervision as a dialogic relationship based in gestalt therapy principles is outlined. Illustrated by examples from a supervisee perspective, themes of 'shame' and the need to attend holistically to the supervisee in their work and personal contexts in the 'here and now', are explored. These examples are discussed in relation to principles of gestalt psychotherapy's concepts of 'contact' and 'liminality'.

Clinical supervisors have an obligation to ensure that the supervisee practises in a way that is 'safe' for the client, themselves and for their employing agencies or professional associations. Supervisors have a further obligation to remain in relationship with the supervisee, as they are engaged in these complex and challenging discussions. The more recent development in the discourse about clinical supervision is the relational emphasis that is discussed in both trauma-informed and gestalt therapy (Clarkson and Aviram, 1995; Hycner and Jacobs, 1995) and applications of concepts such as 'creative adjustment' are applied to clinical supervision (Yontef, 1996). This view enables clinical supervision to be considered as occurring in a liminal space or 'creative void' where learning occurs based on who the supervisee is in the present. Such a view of clinical supervision honours the quality of process and the personhood of the supervisor and supervisee within the inevitable tensions.

How the quality of this relationship supports or constrains the professional development of trauma therapists is explored, drawing from gestalt concepts of inclusion and the dialogic relationship.

## Background

The focus on holism, phenomenology and quality of relationship between the supervisor and supervisee, prevalent in trauma therapy, does not easily fit the reality of clinical supervision offered within many workplaces (Pack, 2012). Increasingly time and financial constraints prevent organizations and individuals from offering what are considered to be the preconditions essential to developing an effective supervisory relationship. These variables include supervision with a trained and experienced supervisor to provide trust and continuity in a clinical supervisory relationship. Within such a relationship, opportunities for engaging in a sustained, on-the-job reflection and dialogue in the 'here and now' from which awareness about practice can grow and flourish over a number of years, is recommended (Clarkson and Aviram, 1995; Cox, 2007). However, this kind of supervisory relationship is an ideal rather than the reality of many practice environments.

Feedback and the way it is given by the clinical supervisor is crucial in establishing the process and relationship. However, the inherent power dynamic of the supervisory relationship militates against supervisees feeling able to express their experiences of clinical supervision openly and honestly, for fear that it might compromise their career or promotional prospects (Chur-Hansen and McLean, 2007; Clarke 1993). This is particularly so when the supervisee is a trainee or new to a field of practice. Deference to the supervisor can be a constraint when supervision occurs in the supervisee's immediate worksite. In this setting the supervisor is generally not chosen by the supervisee, and this is just one of the concerns expressed by clinical supervisees about their experience of clinical supervision (Webb, 2001). Others include the fears of a negative evaluation. This can prevent full disclosure of clinical dilemmas in clinical supervision. A fear of complaints and litigation also militate against such disclosures (Webb, 2001). Another theme involves the mixed roles, functions and agendas encompassed in the concept of clinical supervision. Understanding exactly how the educational, consultative and administrative roles identified for clinical supervision relate to one another can be unclear and is one reason cited for the lack of uptake of clinical supervision despite measures to facilitate access to it (McBride, 2007).

## The many meanings of clinical supervision

In this section I offer a generic definition of clinical supervision and overview two main models of clinical supervision that have been influential in the interdisciplinary literature on clinical supervision. I begin by describing those models that have emerged from an evidence-informed knowledge base and move to discuss how this understanding has been informed by a psychoanalytic and psychodynamic perspective. I will conclude by discussing the influence of gestalt theory on models of clinical supervision and how these models are helpful to ameliorating the vicarious traumatization of trauma therapists.

Clinical supervision has been defined in various ways within different disciplines and models, but is generally considered to be a process of 'guided reflective practice where practitioners share clinical experiences in a structured way to discuss, reflect, evaluate and support one another, providing a forum to maintain and improve standards of care' (Wilson, 1999: 58). Clinical supervision has been aligned with assessment, managerial or monitoring functions, out of which notions of 'professional' or 'clinical' supervision have evolved. To many clinical supervision has come to be regarded as being 'social work's gift to the helping professions' (Wepa, 2007: 13). Managerial supervision has been connected with overseeing, accountability in terms of assessing the performance levels of supervisees in their job functioning, as well as reporting to the professional associations, training agency or employer if practice is unsafe (Hewson, 1992). Key activities include confronting unrecognized feelings or attitudes in the supervisee that are likely to impact on their effectiveness in their work with clients. In contrast, supervisees see the main purpose and task of supervision as being primarily 'educational' and 'supportive' (Cutcliffe and McFeely, 2001; Veeramah, 2002).

The predominant discourse that underlies clinical supervision, derived from the psychoanalytic or psychodynamic framework, is that supervision is a developmental process in which the supervisee gradually learns the necessary skills and confidence required to gain increasing independence from an experienced, knowledgeable clinical supervisor (MacDonald, 2002). However, these definitions lack a sense of coherence and 'fit' to the notion of clinical supervision in trauma work and psychotherapy which also focuses on the process or quality of relationship in clinical supervision (Etherington, 2000). Similarly, the quality of process in clinical supervision has been connected inextricably to good outcomes in clinical supervision from a gestalt psychotherapy perspective (Yontef, 1996). However, this quality of being in clinical supervision and what it means to 'be' in the roles of supervisor and supervisee is a relatively unexplored aspect of the research on clinical supervision (Clarkson and Aviram, 1995). What seems clear about the quality of relationship in clinical supervision is that both supervisor and supervisee are involved in a 'field' or space that is mutually created by the supervisor and supervisee. In this field, context is inseparable from the person and self is experienced in the process of relating to the other (Yontef, 1996). Yontef uses the concept of 'creative adjustment' arising from the paradoxical theory of change to conclude that in clinical supervision, as in all personal therapy 'identifying the actuality of one's existence enables learning and growth' (Yontef, 1996: 94). Conversely, 'trying to change based in disowning who one is, sets up internal dichotomies that stymie growth' (Yontef, 1996: 94). The 'paradoxical theory of change' assumes that staying with the person's truth allows for change to occur and evolve as a natural momentum for change is created by being with the person in the moment.

My understanding is that the 'I–Thou' moment as it is experienced is in some way related to being seen or made present in relation to the other. In clinical supervision, in the 'I–Thou' moment, goals and judgements are temporarily bracketed in this process of attending to the supervisee, and there is a focus on what is happening between the supervisee and the supervisor in the present moment. The 'I–It' realm in clinical supervision concerns the goal of ensuring safe practice by the supervisor's attending to the supervisee in order that the chances of the supervisee meeting the needs of the client in therapy are enhanced. Ideally the 'I–It' and 'I–Thou' moments both exist in the clinical supervisory relationship.

## Examples of 'I–Thou' moments in the clinical supervisory relationship

Gloria, one of the counsellor-participants earlier interviewed, described this 'I–Thou' moment in observing her clinical supervisee, Glenda, who was dealing with the emotional aftermath of a marital break-up while continuing to work part-time as a trauma therapist.

Gloria observed her colleague, Glenda, being personally impacted after a therapy session with clients and felt for her underlying humanity in the difficult situation she was facing at home:

> Gloria: There were a few times when Glenda would come to work and when she would finish a session she would be really, really drained. You could see it. Drained. And we would talk about things. I would be a bit upset for her in that situation that she would have to hear all that stuff and try to do something with it to move on to the next person. So I would feel for her, for Glenda, as a person.

What sometimes disrupts the relationship between clinical supervisor and trauma therapist is the dissociation from the clients they see. This legacy of trauma is often felt secondarily when seeing clients. This response to the work has the potential for beginning to impact the clinical supervisory relationship, in a parallel way.

Douglas, one of the supervisors of the counsellor-participants, discusses his concerns about Kevin, his supervisee who is also a trauma therapist and another of the counsellor-participants interviewed for the vicarious traumatization study. Douglas describes becoming dissociated in observing and assisting his colleague Kevin's dissociative states following Kevin's contact with clients who are also dissociating as they recount their memories of past trauma. Empathetically engaging with Kevin triggered a parallel dissociative state for Douglas supervising Kevin (Pack, 2010).

## A clinical supervisor's perspective

> Douglas: Since I've known Kevin, occasionally I've been worried about Kevin's personal safety, just in terms of his wellness in himself and what he might do with that. I think the dissociation thing, really, if anybody's experiencing (and I know myself from experiencing dissociation in the work that I do with clients), yeah when that's sort of there, it can be very hard to ground people. Sometimes you just have to walk away, give people space and wait for them to get to that point where they can do that themselves. So that's something I do in our relationship.

(Adapted from Pack, 2010)

The addition of the 'I–Thou' process alongside 'I–It' transactions in clinical supervision brings something unique to clinical supervision from a gestalt psychotherapy perspective. The reflection on self and one's practice in the 'here and now' attends to the supervisee's own growth of awareness. Attention in clinical supervision may be on the supervisee's introjects, including those triggered by interactions with clients which may mirror other and perhaps earlier relationships within the supervisee's family of origin. Attention to the supervisee's lively figures and themes are considered important from the supervisee's perspective, yet are missing elements in more task-centred and psychoanalytically based approaches in clinical supervision (Serok and Urda, 1987). While 'I–It' interactions or goal-directed concerns towards purposeful activity are necessary in clinical supervision in relation to team and organizational goals, there is the possibility that these conversations can occur in an environment with an overarching sense of the 'I–Thou' (Buber, 1970), which includes the possibility of a moment of 'illuminated meeting' (Jacobs, 1995: 54). Jacobs sees the 'I–Thou' moment as a 'full-bodied turning toward the other, a surrender to and trust of, the "between"' (1995: 53–4). This relation is seen as residing in the dialogic process that contains the key elements of 'presence, genuine and unreserved communication, and inclusion' (Jacobs, 1995: 64). The notion of 'inclusion' is described as 'the concrete imagining of the reality of the other, in oneself, while still retaining his or her own self-identity' (Jacobs, 1995: 68). Attention to the dialogic relation in gestalt is seen as occurring within 'I–It' or goal-directed interactions. This focus in clinical supervision goes some way to explain the gestalt definition of clinical supervision, as it is described as a process that explores the boundary between the therapist and the client as a way of enlivening the therapeutic process between them. Therefore, what is occurring in clinical supervision has a parallel to what is occurring in the therapeutic relationship. Exploring what is happening in the interface between the therapeutic relationship and the supervisory relationship has the potential for revealing emerging lively figures that all parties can learn from.

I see this 'dialogue' in clinical supervision as occurring in the 'creative void' or holding environment of the supervisory relationship. From this space of 'not knowing' created by the process of the supervisory relationship, insights and awareness can become available. In clinical supervision as in gestalt psychotherapy, there is a balance to be made between support, encouragement and challenge. These three aspects are important for the supervisor to attend to for the personal and professional growth of the supervisee. Ideally, the outcome of this is that supervision can become the place in which 'creative adjustment' can occur, grounded in the paradoxical theory of change (Yontef, 1996). By supporting 'what is', the supervisee's awareness of who they are is honoured, and experimentation with alternative approaches and ways of being can become more available. Yontef (1996) conceptualizes 'creative adjustment' in clinical supervision as a two-way process in which the client–therapist relationship is explored in the process occurring between the supervisor and supervisee. Thus, even in times when these perspectives might conflict, the quality of the relationship and the personhood of the supervisor and supervisee enable exploration of the underlying process that is occurring between supervisor and supervisee as Yontef (1996: 97) suggests:

> The Gestalt therapy supervisor is present as a person, not just an authority – present with warm, authentic and disclosed presence, along with genuine and unreserved communication. It is important that the supervisor's flaws be allowed to show and be acknowledged by the supervisor so that a vertical relationship is not established, i.e. one in which the supervisor is inordinately elevated into having charismatic stature and the supervisee demoted to a lower caste – admiring the supervisor's flawlessness. When the supervisor is present as a person and the supervisees' experience is explicated and respected, then a real dialogue is possible.

## Example: Beth's experience of clinical supervision as a supervisee

Beth, one of the counsellor-participants, was fortunate to have a clinical supervisor over many years with whom her relationship had developed a level of trust in which she was able to disclose how the work was impacting on her in the context of her life, in detail. This enabled Beth to remain centred when dealing with clients who were dissociated and disclosing histories of abuse recently recalled. The supervisory relationship enabled expression of the feelings she had where these feelings could have been internalized and so there was the potential of these responses negatively impacting the relationship with the client. Beth recounted a client who disclosed her childhood abuse to her in a letter as the client was rendered speechless by the shame surrounding her abuse. Beth had a response to the traumatization of her client who was rendered voice-less which was difficult for Beth to articulate due to a parallel process occurring between the therapist and client:

> Beth: I've often had strong reactions … I had a strong reaction to hearing her disclose what happened, a very strong reaction. It came in writing. She couldn't verbalize it in words yet. We both knew there was a lot there to be elicited but she was very, very disso-ciated and a lot of her therapy had been in writing. That was huge for me to hear and read and take in [Beth looks off into space]. So that was an example where I needed to use lots of supervision to deal with that and other ones like that over the years, too, I suppose.

To illuminate what is helpful about this quality of relationship in clinical supervision and its role in the development of psychotherapists and practitioners new to a field of practice, I offer two examples drawn from my earlier experience as a clinical supervisee. These exam-ples are contrasted to a more recent experience of clinical supervision, which exemplifies many of the characteristics of clinical supervision in the ideal description of the gestalt supervisor mentioned by Yontef (1996: 97) as being 'present' as a person.

## Attention to 'figure' and 'ground' in clinical supervision

Prior to entering psychotherapy training, I had two supervisory relationships that exempli-fied two supervisory styles. The first supervisory style was characterized by my supervisor aligning with the administrative functions of supervision. In the first supervisory style, in terms of gestalt therapy principles, I liken this style of supervision to focusing on the supervisor's 'figures' (administrative requirements) while taking the attention from the supervisee's emerging 'figures'. When the conditions of clinical supervision, as defined by the employing organization, are the primary focus, the supervisee's lively figures or issues can be missed, limiting the opportunities for growth and learning in the 'creative void' of the supervisory relationship. In such a relationship, attending to the unknown is not well tolerated, so the supervisee has to 'creatively adjust' to the supervisor being available in a particular way, for example, by being organized primarily around by the requirements of the agency in which they are employed. This style limits the opportunities for the supervisee to explore some of their concerns, uncertainties and the inevitable ambiguities that can arise in the practice environment.

In the second supervisory style I will go on to discuss, the boundaries between personal therapy and clinical supervision were confused. How well supervisors manage the boundary between clinical supervision and personal therapy can impact on the supervisee if the bal-ance is not maintained with the supervisee's practice in mind, or if the personal therapy is not explicitly negotiated or invited by the supervisee.

In gestalt psychotherapy, through the dynamic process of contact, the polarities of isolation and confluence are often prominent. Isolation is described as an experience of detachment from the field of contact whereas confluence involves a merging between the self and other in relationship (Hycner and Jacobs, 1995). On each end of these polarities, there is the possibility of interacting in the space between self and other through a process of one attuning to the other. It is this in-between space that offers opportunities for trust to develop. Trust is the major requirement from a beginning supervisee's perspective for clinical supervision to be considered 'successful' (Serok and Urda, 1987) and from a gestalt psychotherapy perspective. In this way relationship in clinical supervision is connected to 'awareness of awareness' as Hycner and Jacobs (1995) discuss in relation to the relationship between the client and therapist as establishing a dialogic context. In this context, contact can be used to restore connection if it has lapsed, is temporarily lacking or where it has broken down.

On either side of the dialogic process, as each party in the relationship experiments with getting to know the other, isolation and confluence exist as a possibility (Hycner and Jacobs, 1995). Thus, 'the therapist's willingness and receptivity to the sphere of "between" is the scaffolding against which the existential trust of the patient is formed' (Jacobs, 1995: 80). The same polarity can be seen as present in the supervisor–supervisee relationship. Meeting the supervisor at the contact boundary during discussions about defining moments in one's practice risks putting one's actions and view of oneself on the line, raising fears of possible judgement and rejection. If the supervisee feels unmet in the moment in the absence of an attitude of mutual trust, there can be a consequent withdrawal from contact with the other. Restricting the possibilities of contact or meeting the other can lead to a sense of isolation and dissonance. This was the experience with my first supervisor, and is discussed below.

## Supervision as 'isolation'

Clinical supervision in my first two years of practice as a trauma therapist in mental health was conducted with my line manager. She was a team leader, who worked from an apprenticeship model of clinical supervision, in which there was a case-by-case discussion of my planned interventions with each individual client at each session. This focus did not support the development of a relationship that allowed for a fuller discussion of my work. I experienced clinical supervision as a struggle with power and control. These were among the central issues that emerged in my initial experiences of clinical supervision. As I was a younger, less experienced supervisee whose academic achievements were higher than those of my supervisor, in retrospect I believe my academic achievements challenged her sense of authority hence the underlying subtext in our relationship of 'do as I say' and 'remember I'm in charge', which she based on her years of practice. Here was the supervisor who defined my role as being one of unerring compliance for the common good of all. I was reminded in supervision constantly that she was sharing her years of experience with me to save me from what she considered to be my own incompetence. This experience reinforced my negative introjects (which were already well developed). My identification with her judgement that was highly critical of my not being 'good enough', led to cycles of demoralization, shame, retroflection and withdrawal. I felt sure I would be judged negatively for expressing my feelings with her and I believed that this discussion could jeopardize my promotional and career prospects. Thus, I withdrew from much self-disclosure of what was occurring for me from my supervisor, other colleagues and the team. This experience left me feeling disconnected or with a sense of dissonance that compounded the isolation I experienced.

This experience inspired a dread of clinical supervision and undermined rather than enhanced my therapeutic effectiveness. Clinical supervision as a safe refuge from the rigours of practice, a space in which I could reflect upon my practice, seemed unavailable to me. Colleagues in the multidisciplinary team empathized with my position but colluded with the process that remained unresolved until the supervisor's promotion and departure. I recall feeling joyful and triumphant about her leaving as the whole experience felt like an extended status degradation ceremony lasting some three years. The power dynamic inherent in the managerial model of supervision places the supervisee in an impossible bind. The relationship between supervisor and supervisee must always be unequal as the supervisor is empowered to exert power and authority to influence the supervisee's behaviour where the potential risk to the client is ever present. This is in contrast to the therapeutic work of clients that involves supporting the client's process of reclaiming their own power. I now believe, however, that issues of power and control can be acknowledged and creatively explored and worked with, if the quality of relationship in clinical supervision allows for themes of power and control to be more openly discussed between supervisor and supervisee.

Reflecting upon that experience now, I empathize with the supervisor who was struggling to find her voice within the team and was anxious about her professional identity and authority as a new manager. From a relational field perspective, there was no support for the kind of dialogical engagement that would have allowed both of us to explore the process of what was occurring between us, or so it seemed from my perspective. I believe this experience is closely aligned with the issue of 'shame' in the supervisory relationship.

## 'Shame' and the supervisory relationship

In this example, the potential for shame in the supervisory relationship was one of the main issues, as it often is for those new to a field of practice and for those who have not used clinical supervision previously. The potential for shame is often greater where supervised practice is a requirement for professional training or registration (Gill, 2001; Yontef, 1996).

Shame, retroflection and withdrawal can also be issues for more experienced practitioners whose expertise and authority in other fields go unacknowledged. In my experience of teaching and supervising new graduates in mental health, this potential for shame often manifests when key issues are not taken to the supervisory forum. For example, when the supervisee experiences particular knowledge gaps on the job in relation to clients that are unacknowledged by the supervisee, these issues may not be brought for discussion to the supervisory forum. Shame prevents these issues from being taken by the supervisee to supervision in the first place. Further shame results from a felt sense of failure to identify and raise central themes in one's practice in clinical supervision. Trainees who feel ill-prepared to reveal deficits in knowledge may act on their own, thinking that it is preferable to remain independent and not refer to their clinical supervisor. This lack of consultation can result in clinical mishaps such as failing to act appropriately to ensure the safety of clients disclosing suicidal ideation. Such scenarios can cost supervisees their promotional opportunities, and, if unresolved, their jobs. Thus, shame itself can become the central 'issue' that prevents further exploration of the supervisee's experience in clinical supervision. How the shame and guilt evoked in the supervisory process is dealt with remains largely unexplored in the research literature on clinical supervision, however (Alonso and Rutan, 1988; Yontef, 1996).

Another of the ways shame can be evoked in the supervisory relationship is through the process of linking theory and practice. This is particularly so when the supervisee is still in training, and there is a real fear of being exposed as not being able to make these connections (Alonso and Rutan, 1988). In facilitating the application of theory into practice, the clinical supervisor needs to practice 'inclusion' in relation to the supervisee, in much the same way as the therapist does through 'the willingness to enter into the patient's phenomenological world' (Jacobs, 1995: 70). In clinical supervision, inclusion may be demonstrated in the supervisor's ability to be able to feel their way into their supervisee's concerns, identifying shame that might remain unspoken, while being mindful of the need to raise this theme carefully to avoid a flight into further shame, withdrawal and/or confluence.

Shame in the supervisory relationship is more than the opposite of support. The absence of support in clinical supervision is a precondition of the emergence of shame. It is an embarrassment that is often internalized by the supervisee rather than openly expressed for fear of ridicule and humiliation (Alonso and Rutan, 1988). It is best described as 'an experience of disconnectedness characterized by retroflection and withdrawal' (Kearns and Daintry, 2000: 29). The shame that accompanies a revelation of the inadequacy felt by the supervisee to the supervisor under these challenging circumstances can seem all-encompassing. For example, when I encountered as a mental health social worker a situation in which a client's husband continued to contact me about his wife's sessions with me, in which she had disclosed to me confidentially that she was planning to leave him and their marriage, I felt intimidated by his attempts to extract information from me about her. Though I managed the situation by saying that I could not discuss any contact I had had with clients without their consent as this was our agency policy, I felt ashamed of not handling the situation without fear of angry reprisals from family members. I now realize that clinical supervision would have been a useful place to discuss managing therapeutic boundaries and confidentiality to allay the fears I experienced in setting limits. However, I did not feel safe enough to discuss this theme within a managerial style of supervision for fear that it would expose inadequacy and enable my supervisor to judge my practice negatively.

Similarly, the apprenticeship model, prevalent among the teaching of medical professionals, does not translate well to the kinds of clinical supervision favoured by trauma therapists, who prefer to view the process and relationship as more of a collaborative endeavour. Trauma therapists, building on Kadushin's (1992) now classic work on supervision, emphasize the educational purposes of clinical supervision as being underpinned by adult learning principles.

For psychotherapists who work within a gestalt framework in clinical supervision, attention is focused on growing the supervisee's awareness on a number of levels. There is reflection on the self in relationship to the other in terms of the supervisee's exploration of self and interactions in relation to clients in the therapeutic relationship. Second, there is the supervisory forum itself as another space in which to reflect on one's experience in the relationship, as a supervisee in relation to the supervisor. Third, there is awareness of self in relation to the team, colleagues, employing organization and wider social systems representing another layer to be explored in clinical supervision. The process of clinical supervision involves joint reflection on what is happening in the relationship between the supervisor and supervisee, as part of the supervision, on each of these three levels. Consequently, though each practitioner has their own particular style from a gestalt psychotherapy perspective, clinical supervision in gestalt psychotherapy is more strongly weighted towards a process-oriented, multilayered relationship-oriented style than a task-centred approach. Typically, however, there are differences in experience, power and responsibility within the roles of supervisor and supervisor in clinical supervision that are exemplified in the second example of clinical supervision I will now move on to describe.

## Supervision as confluence

The second experience of supervision I want to use as an example occurred in another work context. I was a more mature supervisee, but this time had a supervisor who was a senior colleague/peer, who without contracting to do so, tried to become my therapist. In this supervisory relationship my supervisor assumed the role of wise, all-knowing, guiding supervisor and, as supervisee, I felt cast in the role of a helpless, dependent client. Control was disguised as 'help' and yet therapy was never requested by me or offered explicitly by him in this relationship. I knew that his intention was to 'help' but the affirmation he seemed to seek from me in return, and that I was tacitly agreeing to fulfil, was not what I considered to be the purpose of clinical supervision. I did not question this style of supervision out of a fear of offending or seeming ungrateful. Eventually, after a year in clinical supervision with him I told him that I had found another supervisor outside our immediate team as it was 'time for a change'.

In retrospect my confluence with this process was based on my sense of powerlessness, and my struggle to define the relationship given the differing power positions we held in the organizational hierarchy. My decision to leave the relationship was related to my tiredness of playing the role where I was the recipient of his benevolent 'care'. An example of this attitude was his taking responsibility for bringing along to each session information on personal development courses and 'self-help' literature that he felt would expand my knowledge base on topics unrelated to our previous session. He would use the example of one of his other supervisees having found this approach to his distributing this literature helpful to their personal and career development, but he did not ask for my opinion as to the usefulness of this style from my perspective. I had begun to experience this as an intrusion as I had never explicitly invited nor wished to have therapy disguised as clinical supervision. I longed to be treated collegially by him due to the managerial style of supervision I had earlier experienced and from which I still had not yet fully debriefed. I later found the need to deal with this unfinished business in both supervisory relationships in another forum outside clinical supervision.

Unfortunately, the supervisor did not seem open to a different relationship in clinical supervision, offering instead a fixed form of 'benign benevolence'. When I did leave having found another supervisor, I felt ungrateful and, at the same time, liberated. I had found the contact undermining of my knowledge and skills and so it separated me from the theoretical basis for my work and so also from my resourcefulness and intuitive awareness about myself in my practice.

In the second example, the lack of clear roles and boundaries enabled the exploration of issues in my personal life that were not then related back to practice issues. The power inherent in his role as my supervisor and his senior status in the wider organization left me fearful that I would be judged negatively if I did not demonstrate a receptiveness to his style of supervision (Betcher and Zinberg, 1988). Consequently I felt the kind of vulnerability that comes with the experience of constantly feeling exposed. This situation was compounded by the lack of clarity in terms of the process and structure of clinical supervision, and was underpinned by the power differences between us. It is not an unusual situation for the supervisor and supervisee in an organizational hierarchy. Typically it means that unspoken feelings remain unexpressed, and the risk is that these concerns are internalized by the supervisee as their personal failings. The impact on me was that I felt that I was constantly reminded of what I needed to do to become a more whole person as I was reminded constantly how personal work on the areas identified would improve my progress in my career development. I felt disempowered in my practice and trapped in another's definition of me that seemed to be authored in lack, inadequacy and deficit.

In this example, the clinical supervisor related the 'figures' as he defined them as residing largely in my own therapeutic issues rather than in terms of how they might be impacting on my practice. There was an absence of a particular relational quality that may have allowed us to have a conversation about the impact of his supervisory style with me.

Both styles of clinical supervision I experienced as being unhelpful in developing my practice with clients, as the relationships did not provide the necessary holding or 'liminal' space in which my wider learning and growth could occur. As defined in Chapter 3, liminality is a term used to describe the gap between the known and the unknown, where meaning is attached to experience and in which creative change occurs. Cultural anthropologist

Barbara Myerhoff's classic work *Number Our Days* (1982), building on the earlier work of Turner, uses the concept of entering a 'liminal space' to understand the process of adjustment experienced by migrants entering into a new culture who meet to share narratives of the 'old country' from the new (Myerhoff, 1982). When self and other interact in such spaces, new life-enhancing narratives and meanings are created (Myerhoff, 1982). I have conceptualised 'liminal' spaces as existing when practitioners move to a new field of practice and are challenged to evolve their own styles and ways of working with complex themes and issues. This process of developing new ways of transitioning to a new field parallels a movement from one culture to another (Pack, 2004, 2007). Within such discursive spaces, individual practitioners experience an immersion in the unknown that is akin to the 'creative void' or 'impasse'. Out of this, creative void strategies and solutions to challenges are actively evolved through interaction of the self within the practice environment, and through professional associations (Pack, 2004, 2007). Clinical supervision itself represents a liminal zone of 'betwixt and between' in which clinical dilemmas and puzzles can be deliberated on and experimentation with new strategies and ways of being can be evolved and tested for relevance and meaning in cycles of action and reflection. Regardless of whether the practitioner is new to a field, one could argue that clinical supervision offers an opportunity to step into the unknown and so provides opportunities to interact in liminal spaces at whatever phase in career development. Therefore, this concept has relevance and its understanding can be extended to apply to more experienced practitioners as well as newcomers to the field of practice. In trauma-related psychotherapy, as Beth, Douglas, Kevin, Gloria and Glenda's narratives attest in this and previous chapters, clinical supervision, to be effective, relies on the quality of relationship that attends empathetically to the whole person.

## The dialogic relationship in clinical supervision

As a consequence of these experiences in clinical supervision, I valued increasingly a supervisory process that functioned more as a 'dialogical relationship' (Hycner and Jacobs, 1995). What I understand this to mean is that attention is paid to the practice of inclusion and there is a cultivation of the dialogic to provide the 'ground' for the relationship in clinical supervision. By attending to 'what is' through a process of dialogical engagement, new directions and ways of being in the supervisee's practice become available (Pack, 2009b).

Defined in this way, the dialogic relationship can be seen as providing a liminal space or 'creative void'. This space supports the safe exploration of existential themes, uncertainty and complexity. Though each therapist has a different interpretation of the supervisory relationship, supervision for gestalt therapists has an overarching 'oral tradition' in which a number of key principles guide practice (Yontef, 1996). These principles include inclusion, awareness of the awareness process, and personal and professional growth through the supervisory process and relationship. Through the establishment of the supervisory relationship as a dialogic forum where a sense of the 'I–Thou' develops can be facilitated and grown from 'I–It' discussions, a liminal or holding space is created. This occurs because the individual supervisee, when faced by various on-the-job challenges, needs a forum to make meaning of new experience, and to relate what is known already to the new situation that is being explored. This process enables the supervisee to evolve actions and attach meaning to experience for the future. In this way, a reservoir of practice wisdom, based in experience, can be grown in the process of clinical supervision when it is working well for both supervisee and supervisor. The supervisor in clinical supervision, ideally, is genuine, present and available to witness this process which is parallel to the growth of awareness that occurs in the client–therapist relationship over time. When the relationship in clinical supervision attends to the process occurring between the supervisor and supervisee, this provides transparency and fosters trust. This trust opens a space within which conversations based in awareness can develop more easily. Within this space, which I liken to the 'creative void', the 'inward eye' or awareness of self in the practice environment can develop. Erskine (1982) describes this as the capacity for multiple levels of simultaneous awareness within supervision, and the ability of a 'shuttling' process backwards and forwards between the processes occurring between client and therapist and supervisor and supervisee. Thus, 'it is this ability to be in contact with one's own internal experience and the uniqueness of the client's experience that is the basis for empathy' (Erskine, 1982: 316). This 'inner eye' could also describe an awareness of the co-created field between the supervisor and supervisee and, as such, create the 'ground' of the supervisory relationship. It is the process of becoming cognizant of 'our awareness of the awareness process' within clinical supervision (Yontef, 1996: 92). This capacity for the dialogical principle of inclusion within clinical supervision is a level of support that mitigates against the emergence of shame and this then allows for more of this challenging inquiry to develop. This is the process by which supervisees grow in their own awareness. Ultimately, the discernment of the 'inner eye' or the development of the internal supervisor within the supervisee connects the influence of supervision in psychotherapy with being therapeutic with clients by freeing up the resources of the supervisee to enable them to support the client's process more fully (Pack, 2009b).

## Supervision as a liminal space

My most positive experience of clinical supervision was with a supervisor who was a psychotherapist by training. The relationship we created together enabled me to freely disclose the emotional impact of my work with clients without fear of recrimination in the organizational structure. As she was externally employed rather than a work colleague, she offered a fresh perspective on the material I brought to clinical supervision. Her positioning outside my employment facilitated a non-hierarchical relationship in which we were able to engage in a process of negotiation within a climate of mutual trust and respect. Through a process that was transparent to me and in which I had an equal voice, she facilitated discussion of issues on the three aspects of my practice that involved my relationship and practice with clients, with colleagues and the team, and with her as part of the relationship in clinical supervision. When I felt weary and defeated at times in the complexities of the workplace, she offered an attitude of optimism about and for my practice, which focused on my resourcefulness and knowledge. Her self-disclosure of her own practice experiences allowed me to see her as fully present and attentive and human without the professional superiority of my first supervisor or the intrusiveness of the second. Her style as supervisor in clinical supervision opened the way to genuine meeting and creative possibilities from my perspective. This style of clinical supervision nurtured my awareness of myself in my practice and allowed me to more confidently function in my work with clients due to the balance of challenge and support provided in the clinical supervision relationship and facilitated by the personal qualities of the supervisor.

---

### Questions for reflection

Thinking about your experiences in clinical supervision:

- What is 'good' clinical supervision from your experience?
- Do you have a quiet, regular time to meet with a clinical supervisor where you can reflect in an unhurried, reflective way about your work, career goals and themes in your work?
- Do you have a trusting, respectful relationship with your clinical supervisor? To consider this question you might like to reflect on how you feel after your supervision session. Do you actively plan and look forward to your clinical supervision?
- If not, consider how you can begin to get the supervision that will support you in your work as a trauma therapist. See the resources at the end of this chapter for initial ideas.
- Begin by consulting your professional association and colleagues for ideas about where to go and how to obtain quality clinical supervision within a respectful relationship with a clinical supervisor.

---

## Maintaining relationship

The dialogic approach is recommended when dealing with trauma disclosures (Etherington, 2000). A focus based in the 'I–Thou' relationship mitigates against shame and so this process is less likely to evoke the polarity of confluence and isolation that can be seen as existing on either side of this process and is exemplified in the two styles of clinical supervision described from my experience. The development of a relationship in clinical supervision is evoked where greater transparency is likely.

These experiences suggest the need for balance between the 'I–Thou' and 'I–It' or goal-directed processes in clinical supervision. There are supervisory styles and processes that are more conducive to evoking each side of the confluence–isolation polarity in my experience, depending on how supervisors and supervisees define their relationship and meet one another in clinical supervision. The supervisee's and supervisor's respective definitions and meanings of clinical supervision can be quite dissimilar and so becoming acquainted with the 'other' is necessary at the outset of the relationship (Pack, 2009b).

Supervisees in beginning supervision or those changing professions can struggle with shame in getting to know the other of the supervisor. In this process, the supervisee risks becoming enmeshed in a cycle of shame producing further shame which one of my trainers in gestalt psychotherapy referred to as 'going down the shame drain'. Triggers to shame reactions may be located in earlier supervisory or team relationships. These relationships and the supervisee's past experiences within them may become figural when shame is evoked. Shame may have a further basis in unresolved family-of-origin dynamics. Shame may be the underlying yet lively figure in the supervisory forum and require attention in clinical supervision and/or in personal therapy.

There are a number of key prerequisites for cultivating the environment in which the supervisee's awareness can grow and flourish. These conditions involve the establishment of the 'dialogic attitude' based in the principle of inclusion (Yontef, 1996). This dialogical attitude helps to create a space where the inevitable power differential between supervisor and supervisee (especially within an organizational hierarchy) can be acknowledged and worked with usefully.

To establish safety and to avoid unintended intrusions of privacy and shaming, there needs to be a clear, mutual understanding and explicit boundary about the interface between supervision and personal therapy. In training and fieldwork supervision where academic assessment is required, this function also needs to be made explicit and open for ongoing discussion and debate. Safety of the supervisee and client, the boundaries of confidentiality, and privacy need also to be part of the dialogue, as does an understanding about the purpose of supervision. Such mutual understanding is critical yet usually untested until there is a 'problem' identified, and often this is identified too late to be processed within the clinical supervision relationship (Pack, 2009b).

In summary, clinical supervision is a learning experience for the supervisee and supervisor – a mutual journey of discovery. If the supervisor is working from a shared understanding of the purpose and process of supervision, there is a frame of reference or 'ground' from which each can relate to the other. If the supervisor can provide a 'creative void' or liminal space and keep it available, where 'not knowing' is valued, much learning is possible. If the supervisor has the capacity to model the holding of faith and trust necessary for the dialogic relationship to be there, the supervisee's capacity for empathy and use of the whole self with clients in therapy is enhanced. The practice of the dialogic relationship in supervision can support the supervisee/therapist in their process of trusting in their own becoming. This is one of the challenges that the supervisory relationship presents, and something a dialogical approach makes possible.

## Checklist for core components of effective clinical supervision

- A trusting, mutually respectful relationship between supervisor and supervisee that is confidential.
- A clear contract or agreement about how you will use the time in supervision, including you and your supervisor's responsibilities.
- A regular time to meet with a shared agenda and responsibilities.
- A quiet, pleasant meeting venue in which to reflect and uninterrupted time.
- A supervisor who ideally is not your line manager as these roles generally need to be kept separate to ensure that the boundaries are clear between performance appraisal and clinical supervision.
- A focus on the dynamics of the therapeutic relationship, including countertransference and traumatic transference in the therapist–client and in the therapist–supervisor relationships.
- Knowledge about the ongoing effects of vicarious traumatization and the need for education about the ongoing impact of the work on a regular updated basis.
- A supervisor who has knowledge of multi-theoretical frameworks for practice, including trauma-informed theory, psychodynamic theory, dissociation and other trauma-related presentations.
- Supervision that allows discussion of the interface between professional and personal issues in relation to how the work is impacting at home.
- A focus on the organization and colleague relationships that affect the work, particularly where the agency's focus is on trauma and trauma recovery.

## Reformulated understandings of clinical supervision across the multidisciplines

More recent developments in the themes behind clinical supervision have been related to how the client–therapist relationship is re-enacted within the supervisory relationship (Pack, 2009a, 2009b). The parallel process of developing a working relationship with one's clinical supervisor is discussed in the research literature in relation to maintaining effective therapeutic relationships with one's clients (Mazzetti, 2007).

Patterns of interaction or the 'games played' by the supervisor and supervisee in clinical supervision have been associated with the supervisor's efforts to resolve conflicts with asserting their authority and the supervisee's confluence with the process (Hawthorne, 1992, building on the work of Kadushin, 1992). These dynamics in clinical supervision can become fixed in the supervisory process over time, acting to derail its effectiveness. Although refusal to 'play the game' and to decide to 'name the game' is the way out of such fixed gestalts or patterns of relating, often the supervisee is in too vulnerable a position to admit that there is a problem through confrontation (Hawthorne, 1992). These dynamics in clinical supervision can stem from a variety of factors, including the supervisor and supervisee's differing positioning and power in the organizational hierarchy and the nature of the interaction between them. Each may be working from different theories and understandings of clinical supervision due to their divergent experiences (Landmark *et al.*, 2003).

## Insights from transactional analysis (TA)

Many of the generic principles underlying transactional analysis (TA) theory and practice when applied to the relationship in clinical supervision are useful to trauma therapists' underlying concern with social justice principles. These concepts include equal relationship, open communication and negotiation, contracting to establish process, and revisiting each participant's understanding of the contract in an adult-to-adult rather than adult-to-child interaction. In TA models, the linkages within the client–supervisor–supervisee 'triad' are illuminated as the contract between the worker and the client is also revisited for relevance. Therefore, the focus is one that 'remembers to put the choices back with the client' as they are modelled in the relationship between the supervisee and supervisor in clinical supervision. (Cox, 2007: 105).

Mazzetti (2007), from a TA perspective, building upon the models of Erskine (1982) and Clarkson (1992), divides the emotional experiences encountered by the supervisee in clinical supervision as those related to the inner dialogue of the supervisee, and countertransference within the supervisee–supervisor–client triad. He argues that in the beginning phase, supervisees require 'protection' in supervision as their enthusiasm increases the likelihood that they will take on too much work-wise and become overloaded (Mazzetti, 2007). The potential for vicarious traumatization, burnout and compassion fatigue, therefore, features prominently in this phase of the trauma therapist's professional career development.

Later in the supervisee's development, the focus needs to be more on the transferential issues in terms of increasing the supervisee's awareness of issues that they may be unconsciously projecting onto clients (Mazzetti, 2007). Fundamental to this model is the supervisor's modelling of the supervisory process by developing a relationship involving TA concepts of 'I'm OK – you're OK' based in an adult-to-adult interaction, contracting and an awareness of 'parallel process' or patterns in the supervisory relationship mirroring the relationship between the client and supervisee (Mazzetti, 2007). In such a relationship, shifts in the supervisee's cognitive constructs, belief and value systems and frames of reference (characteristic of the development of vicarious traumatization) can be more openly explored in clinical supervision.

## Preconditions for 'good supervision' and the developmental needs of supervisees

It is acknowledged in the majority of studies on clinical supervision that without trust and respect, the supervisory relationship will be unlikely to provide the sense of safety and protection necessary for the depth of reflection and awareness to unfold (Cerinus, 2005). Trust and safety balanced with challenge are preconditions that are necessary for the supervisory relationship to work and to maximize its effectiveness from the supervisee's perspective (Cerinus, 2005; Kolade, 2005; Lingren *et al.*, 2005). For example, in the first 12 months of practice, one action research study found that trust was seen by supervisees as being an essential component of empathy and if it was not present there was little chance of an effective working relationship (Cerinus, 2005). Without these preconditions of safety and trust, supervision is unable to be truly effective and becomes instead 'disabling and restrictive' (Cutcliffe and McFeely, 2001: 315). These findings mirror those meanings supervisees attribute to 'effective' clinical supervision (Clarkson and Aviram, 1995). As trust in relationships more generally may be affected by vicarious traumatization, trust-building is particularly relevant for considering within the clinical supervisory relationship.

Choice of supervisor and an environment of trust and confidence in the first year are necessary for an effective supervisory relationship, with challenge being considered less important for newer supervisees (Cutcliffe and McFeely, 2001). On a similar theme, another qualitative study of counselling supervision using a grounded theory methodology from the supervisee's viewpoint, identifies the importance of 'safety' or 'a safe relationship' in which the supervisee's chosen model of working is understood by the supervisor (Weaks, 2002). The 'equality' of relationship is considered enhanced by 'shared beliefs and values' between supervisor and supervisee (Weaks, 2002: 37). Within such a supervisory relationship, challenge is seen as being necessary for clinical supervision to be considered a meaningful experience by the counsellor-participants interviewed (Weaks, 2002).

## Being a clinical supervisee

Increasingly, evaluative studies have been undertaken from the supervisees' perspective with a focus on the quality of the supervisory relationship. For example, one phenomenological study of supervisees' experience of clinical supervision concluded that 'providing support, facilitating growth, enhancing and enriching practice safety and encountering a fresh experience' were the key themes from semi-structured interviews conducted with five focus groups (Cutcliffe and McFeely, 2001: 314).

Jones (1998) researched the role of supervision for oncology nurses working with the terminally ill and discovered that there were deeper existential realities revealed for supervisees through their extended reflection on their practice in the clinical supervisory relationship. Building on Yalom's (1989) work, the author concludes that realizing tacit practices through reflection on practice has the potential to grow expertise professionally and personally through a 'boundary experience' in which the clinician's core values and life experiences become integrated with their practice through reflection in clinical supervision (Jones, 1998).

## Being a clinical supervisor

The unavailability of adequate time to build rapport and attend to the supervisees' needs adequately, coupled with confusion over roles and responsibilities, continue to be discussed in relation to the supervisor's perspective of clinical supervision (Saarikoski *et al.*, 2007). The efficacy of supervisors to effectively balance a complexity of tasks and roles simultaneously is highlighted in the supervisory literature (Banks, 1975). Supervisors can feel torn between the needs of the organization, supervisees and clients. They endeavour to function as role models to supervisees yet struggle to establish an equal relationship in the process of clinical supervision as they are required to exert their authority to manage (Landmark *et al.*, 2003).

Two specific styles of supervisors have been identified in a study of nursing supervisors in clinical supervision. The 'emotional' style pertains more to creating a relationship and dialogue to support the supervisee, and the 'cognitive' style reflects the supervisor's ability to apply theory for assisting the supervisee to problem-solve in practice scenarios (Severinsson and Hallberg, 1996: 155–6). Personal qualities considered important for supervisors are 'willingness and preparedness to show understanding, bringing out genuine feelings, confirming and being sensitive to the supervisees' needs' (Severinsson and Hallberg, 1996: 156). The judicious use of self-disclosure by the supervisor and a focus on reflection on practice are considered to be among the essential skills for the clinical supervisor to develop (Wilson, 1999).

## Feedback and critique

Availability and the way that feedback is given by supervisors in clinical supervision are considered important variables in the effectiveness of clinical supervision from the supervisee's perspective. Giving and receiving clear feedback through a regular supervisory contact that is empathetic is preferred by supervisees (Chur-Hansen and McLean, 2007; Heckman-Stone, 2003). A pilot study of trainee preferences for feedback in trauma therapists found that supervisees preferred supervisors who were flexible in their use of theoretical models, confident in their abilities and who avoided taking on the role of therapist (Heckman-Stone, 2003). 'Constructive feedback' delivered in a timely manner built confidence in the practitioner's use of their discretion and clinical reasoning (Heckman-Stone, 2003).

Improving supervisors' skills to provide formative feedback more consistently and effectively from within current teaching and learning theories is much recommended across the disciplines (Chur-Hansen and McLean, 2007; Macdonald, 2002; Saarikoski *et al.*, 2007). One of the main obstacles in implementing these recommendations is supervisors' lack of confidence in giving feedback, coupled with fears of complaints and litigation (Chur-Hansen and McLean, 2007).

## The implications from the literature for establishing clinical supervision as a forum for critical reflection

Confusion over how to distinguish the differences between appraisal, performance management and clinical supervision as reflection on and for practice is a recurring theme in the literature (Sexton-Bradshaw, 1999). Among the many meanings attributed to clinical supervision, it is seen as a self-management strategy and as a way of ameliorating the stress of the day-to-day work. Other purposes are to increase self-awareness in one's practice and to enhance the therapeutic value of one's work with clients (Begat *et al.*, 2005). The difficulty with these mixed roles and meanings is that they remain tacit and so the functioning of management and clinical models/roles are inherently in conflict. One key dilemma for supervisors is the role they are required to fulfil in acting as a teacher, mentor, educator and role model simultaneously.

## Recommendations to inform workplace action

Choice of supervisor by the supervisee is considered universally important with supervision offered for a trial four-to-six-week period recommended for supervisees (Sexton-Bradshaw, 1999). For beginning trauma therapists, frequency of meeting is an issue, as feedback needs to be given in a more systematic way to develop practice at the beginning of one's career. For more experienced practitioners, clinical supervision on the strategic development of one's career through a focus on short- and longer-term professional development objectives is recommended (Mazzetti, 2007). Factors such as time and adequate training of supervisors need to be taken into account in the resourcing of clinical supervision within agency contexts, to allow the supervisory relationship to develop, acknowledging the realities and pragmatic constraints. Training about clinical supervision for both supervisees and supervisors is discussed in this paper with reference to a range of models in which supervision is depicted as more than a concept but instead as an 'overarching philosophy for professional practice' (Wilson, 1999: 58). In this training, Mothersole's (1998) model of clinical supervision, which is derived from a transactional analysis model, establishes a process and structure that attends to the micro-level of the session and identifies themes in supervisees' practice over time. This model considers the clients', supervisors' and supervisees' socio-economic position, work setting, class, culture and ethnicity. This type of multilevel approach enables supervisors to attend to the supervisee's personal well-being, their practice, as well as workload and case mix, and the interpersonal dynamics in clinical supervision between supervisor and supervisee. The wider social systems of client and supervisor–supervisee and their employing agencies can be explored within this type of multilevel approach.

## Conclusion

Supervisees in beginning supervision or those who move fields of practice can struggle with shame and disconnection in getting to know the 'other' of the supervisor in clinical supervision. In this process, the supervisee risks becoming enmeshed in a cycle of fear, producing further shame and withdrawal. This disconnection can affect clients' and supervisees' well-being (Pack, 2009a, 2009b).

There are a number of key prerequisites for cultivating the environment in which the supervisee's awareness can grow and flourish. These conditions involve the establishment of a relationship in which the inevitable tensions and power differential between supervisor and supervisee can be acknowledged and discussed. When the supervisory relationship is conceptualized in this way, it has a greater potential for establishing clinical supervision as a co-created space in which a sustained reflection on practice can occur from a mutual understanding of process and a shared experience of learning. This process involves a clear purpose and contract for how the relationship in clinical supervision will operate, establish how and when feedback will be given, and the effectiveness of the relationship will be reviewed and evaluated. The supervisory contract requires strategies to maintain connection, to negotiate difference and plan for the inevitable disconnections that occur in relationships. Supervisors need to have an awareness of the purpose of their role, to be adequately prepared and trained to validate and find empathetic ways to offer constructive critique of their supervisees' practice in ways that avoid shaming and humiliation.

In conclusion, this chapter, based on a systematic literature review, interviews with trauma counsellors and personal insights, provides support for clinical supervision to be guided by the same process and elements of any growth-fostering relationship. These elements include open and transparent communication and process, trust, safety, mutuality, equal voice, free disclosure, and regular and timely feedback. Within the supervisory relationship, clinical supervision represents a holding space in which the supervisor works with the faith that the relationship created will foster the resilience and personal and professional growth for supervisees that will, in turn, enable a parallel process of growth to occur with the supervisee's clients. To achieve these aims, clinical supervision needs to be more formally recognized and embedded in the organizational philosophy for it to be 'successful' for both supervisor and supervisee. Only then will supervisees have the confidence to use clinical supervision effectively and supervisors will have the mandate to use the time and resources provided to demonstrate and model its usefulness within the organizational framework. In the following chapter, we consider how the organization provides for the needs of trauma therapists with clinical supervision as one of a range of strategies supporting self-care.

## Weblinks and resources

### For clinical supervisors

Australian Clinical Supervisors' Association:

http://clinicalsupervision.org.au

Conference monograph on advances in clinical supervision:

New South Wales Institute of Psychiatry. (2013). Advances in clinical supervision: Innovation and practice – a selection of papers presented at the Advances in Clinical Supervision Conference, Sydney, Australia, 4–6 June. Retrieved from: www.nswiop.nsw.edu.au/images/publications/clinsup-monograph.pdf (accessed 1 March 2016).

National Association of Social Workers. (2013). *Best standards in social work supervision*. Retrieved from: www.naswdc.org/practice/naswstandards/supervisionstandards2013.pdf (accessed 1 March 2016).

New South Wales Institute of Psychiatry:

www.nswiop.nsw.edu.au

### For clinical supervisees

To find a new supervisor these websites may be helpful to consult:

http://adelaidetraumacentre.com.au/professional-support/clinical-supervision
http://changehappens.com.au/services/clinical-supervision

# References

Alonso, A. and Rutan, S. (1988). Shame and guilt in psychotherapy supervision. *Psychotherapy, 25* (4), 576–81.

Banks, B. (1975). On being a supervisor. *Supervisor Nurse, 6* (8), 19–20.

Begat, I., Ellefsen, B. and Severinsson, E. (2005). Nurses' satisfaction with their work environment and the outcome of clinical nursing supervision on nurses' experiences of well-being: A Norwegian study. *Journal of Nursing Management, 13* (3), 221–30.

Betcher, R. W. and Zinberg, N. E. (1988). Supervision and privacy in psychotherapy training. *American Journal of Psychiatry, 145* (7), 796–803.

Buber, M. (1970). *I and Thou.* New York: Charles Scribner's Sons.

Cerinus, M. (2005). The role of relationships in effective clinical supervision. *Nursing Times, 101* (14), 34–7.

Chur-Hansen, A. and McLean, S. (2007). Trainee psychiatrists' views about their supervisors and supervision. *Australasian Psychiatry, 15* (4), 269–72.

Clarke, D. M. (1993). Supervision in the training of a psychiatrist. *Australian and New Zealand Journal of Psychiatry, 27* (2), 306–10.

Clarkson, P. (1992). *Transactional analysis psychotherapy: An integrated approach.* London: Routledge.

Clarkson, P. and Aviram, O. (1995). Phenomenological research on supervision: Supervisors reflect on 'being a supervisor'. *Counselling Psychology Quarterly, 8* (1), 63–80.

Cox, M. (2007). On doing supervision. *Transactional Analysis Journal, 37* (2), 104–14.

Cutcliffe, J. and McFeely, S. (2001). Practice nurses and their 'lived experience' of clinical supervision. *British Journal of Nursing, 10* (5), 312–23.

Erskine, R. (1982). Supervision of psychotherapy: Models for professional development. *Transactional Analysis Journal, 12* (4), 314–21.

Etherington, K. (2000). Supervising counsellors who work with survivors of childhood sexual abuse. *Counselling Psychology Quarterly, 13* (4), 377–89.

Gill, S. (2001). *The supervisory alliance: Facilitating the psychotherapist's learning experience.* Lanham, MD: Jason Aronson.

Hawthorne, L. (1992). *Games supervisors play.* Dunedin, NZ: Department of Extension, Otago University.

Heckman-Stone, C. (2003). Trainee preferences for feedback and evaluation in clinical supervision. *Clinical Supervisor, 22* (1), 21–33.

Hewson, D. (1992). Supervising counsellors. *The Australian Counselling Psychologist, 8* (1), 9–22.

Hycner, R. and Jacobs, L. (1995). *The healing relationship in gestalt therapy: A dialogic/self psychology approach.* New York: Gestalt Journal.

Jacobs, L. (1995). Dialogue in gestalt theory and therapy. In Hycner, R. and Jacobs, L., *The healing relationship in gestalt therapy: A dialogic/self psychology approach* (pp. 51–84). New York: Gestalt Journal.

Jones, A. (1998). Clinical supervision with community Macmillan nurses: Some theoretical suppositions and case work reports. *European Journal of Cancer Care, 7* (1), 63–9.

Kadushin, A. (1992). *Supervision in social work* (3rd edn). New York: Columbia University Press.

Kearns, A. and Daintry, P. (2000). Shame in the supervisory relationship: Living with the enemy. *British Journal of Gestalt, 9* (1), 28–38.

Kolade, S. T. (2005). Nurses' perception of clinical supervision. *West African Journal of Nursing, 16* (1), 11–19.

Landmark, B. T., Hansen, G. S., Bjones, I. and Bohler, A. (2003). Clinical supervision: Factors defined by nurses as influential upon the development of competence and skills in supervision. *Journal of Clinical Nursing, 12* (6), 834–41.

Lindgren, B., Brulin, C., Holmlund, K. and Athlin, E. (2005). Nursing students' perception of group supervision during clinical training. *Journal of Clinical Nursing, 14* (7), 822–9.

McBride, P. (2007). Clinical supervision and the use of structured homework. *Mental Health Practice, 10* (6), 29–30.

MacDonald, J. (2002). Clinical supervision: A review of underlying concepts and developments. *Australian and New Zealand Journal of Psychiatry, 36* (1), 92–8.

Mazzetti, M. (2007). Supervision in transactional analysis: An operational model. *Transactional Analysis Journal, 37* (2), 93–103.

Mothersole, G. (1998). Levels of attention in clinical supervision. *Transactional Analysis Journal, 28* (4), 299–310.

Myerhoff, B. G. (1982). *Number our days: Triumph of continuity and culture among Jewish old people in an urban ghetto.* New York: Simon & Schuster/Touchstone Books.

Pack, M. J. (2004). Sexual abuse counsellors' responses to stress and trauma: A social work perspective. *New Zealand Journal of Counselling, 25* (2), 1–17.

Pack, M. J. (2007). The concept of hope in gestalt therapy: Its usefulness for ameliorating vicarious traumatisation. *Gestalt Australia and New Zealand Journal, 3* (25), 59–71.

Pack, M. (2009a). Clinical supervision: An interdisciplinary review of literature with implications for reflective practice in social work. *Reflective Practice, 10* (5), 657–68.

Pack, M. (2009b). Supervision as a liminal space: Towards a dialogic relationship. *Gestalt Journal of Australia and New Zealand, 5* (2), 60–78.

Pack, M. (2010). Career themes in the lives of sexual abuse counsellors. *New Zealand Journal of Counselling, 30* (2), 75–92.

Pack, M. (2012). Vicarious traumatisation: An organisational perspective. *Social Work Now: The Practice Journal of Child, Youth and Family, 50,* 14–23.

Pack, M. J. (2015). Unsticking the stuckness: A qualitative study of the clinical supervisory needs of early career health social workers. *British Journal of Social Work, 45* (6), 1821–36. doi: 10.1093/bjsw/bcu069

Saarikoski, M., Marrow, C., Abreu, W., Riklikiene, O. and Ozbicakci, S. (2007). Student nurses' experience of supervision and mentorship in clinical practice: A cross cultural perspective. *Nurse Education in Practice, 7* (6), 407–15.

Serok, S. and Urda, L. V. (1987). Supervision in social work from a gestalt perspective. *Clinical Supervisor, 5* (2), 69–85.

Severinsson, E. I. and Hallberg, I.R. (1996). Clinical supervisors' views of their role in the process within nursing care. *Journal of Advanced Nursing, 24* (1), 151–161. doi: 10.1046/j.1365-2648.1996.17321.x

Sexton-Bradshaw, D. (1999). Nurses' perceptions of the value of clinical supervision. *Paediatric Nursing, 11* (3), 34–7.

Veeramah, V. (2002). The benefits of using clinical supervision. *Mental Health Nursing, 22* (1), 18–23.

Weaks, D. (2002). Unlocking the secrets of 'good supervision': A phenomenological exploration of experienced counsellors' perceptions of good supervision. *Counselling and Psychotherapy Research, 2* (1), 33–9.

Webb, A. (2001). Honesty in supervision. *Counselling and Psychotherapy Journal, 12* (5), 24–5.

Wepa, D. (Ed). (2007). *Clinical supervision in Aotearoa/New Zealand: A health perspective.* Auckland: Pearson Education New Zealand.

Wilson, J. (1999). Clinical supervision: Practicalities for the supervisor. *Accident and Emergency Nursing, 7* (1), 58–64.

Yalom, I. D. (1989). *Love's executioner and other tales of psychotherapy.* New York: Basic Books.

Yontef, G. (1996). Supervision from a gestalt therapy perspective. *British Gestalt Journal, 5* (2), 92–102.

# Chapter 6    **Vicarious traumatization**

## An organizational perspective

My worst thing is writing those intensive reports [assessment and treatment plans required for sensitive claim cover]. When I have to write without being in relationship to them [survivor clients] I'm writing about them and somehow that's the worst for me. I haven't worked out quite why it's such a terrible thing. Sometimes I've just got to walk away or I'd sit there and yell at the reports I am writing! [exasperated laugh]. What's been done and such, you know, that's really a lot of what the intensive reports are reporting – events that are quite cruel and violent as well as sexual. [gap, when I pause the tape as Angela's eyes fill with tears. The recorded interview continues at her request.] I find that, that traumatic [voice trails off in a moment of self-reflection].

*Angela, one of the counsellor-participants talking about writing the in-depth assessment and treatment plans for ACC and how this organizational requirement affects her well-being*

## Introduction

In this chapter, the stress and trauma experienced by sexual abuse counsellors is explored with implications for promoting effective teamwork within organizations.

As outlined in the previous chapters, therapists who work with adult survivors in the trauma field have a strong preference for working within narrative, strengths-based and emancipatory theoretical approaches (Pack, 2004). The relevance of 'vicarious traumatization' (i.e. the impact on trauma therapists of sharing their clients' feelings and trauma) and self-development theories are central to trauma therapists' self-care and well-being. Current literature about vicarious traumatization suggests that the experience of vicarious traumatization compounds with exposure to their clients' trauma if appropriate self-care strategies are not in place (Rabu *et al.*, 2015). Where the team and organizational functioning does not support therapists' self-care measures formally, this lack of alignment of personal and professional self-care strategies increases or amplifies the risk of burnout and secondary traumatization on the worker (Pack, 2012). In terms of organizational support strategies to ameliorate and prevent vicarious traumatization, the need for continuing research into the impact of supervision, training, teamwork and consultation has been highlighted in a recent systemic review of the literature on vicarious traumatization among practitioners who work with sexual violence and child sexual abuse (Chouliara *et al.*, 2009). Therefore, any new therapists entering organizations dealing with trauma need to be alerted to possible effects and hazards at the outset of the recruitment and appointment process to the employing organization.

In this way, research undertaken internationally has found that counsellors', social workers' or other helping professionals' responses to their clients' trauma are further amplified by the nature of organizational frameworks that surround them in their practice (van Heugten, 1999, 2011). The practice frameworks therapists work under are, at times, at odds with the philosophies of the agencies within which they practise, causing tension and an increased risk of secondary and vicarious traumatization (Pack, 2004). For example, the initial assessment of sexual abuse recovery primarily takes place in medico-legal environments. Subsequently, survivors are referred or self-refer to therapists approved to provide this service under public funding contracts. When the funding and organizational reporting requirements are 'top down' and managerially prescribed, which is often emphasized when restructuring or economic retrenchment in the health and welfare sectors occurs, trauma therapists become akin to change managers on behalf of their employing or contracting organizations. Through the use of their discretion by the interpretation of policy and even in relation to the way in which they report what clients tell them in assessment and treatment reports, decisions about eligibility for service are made. This managerial model required by many bureaucratic organizations relies on the human service workers to operationalize and deliver services that align with these policies and processes that are very often driven by budgetary factors. This approach contrasts with the ways in which trauma therapists prefer to work (Pack, 2012). Trauma therapy, from the counsellor-participants' perspectives, most often drew from narrative, rights-based and anti-oppressive paradigms in which the therapeutic relationship is conceptualized as a co-created space in which the hierarchical or 'expert-knows-best' positioning of the counsellor in relation to clients is reformulated (Pack, 2004).

Legal and medically based agencies who work alongside therapists with trauma survivors often rely on formal types of assessment and forensic investigation which happen in a series of time-framed interventions outside the control of the client and therapist. This kind of environment can stifle the therapist's sense of control and autonomy which, as we have seen in Chapter 1, are key factors in contributing to the burnout and compassion fatigue of trauma-related work. As a consequence, within the context of multidisciplinary teams, trauma therapists sometimes report experiencing a sense of dissonance in the helping endeavour due to their differing approaches to practice and theoretical paradigms. Trauma therapy is congruent with an emancipatory, narrative, social justice paradigm, where the therapist works collaboratively with clients to focus on fostering autonomy and self-determination in the therapeutic process (Pack, 2010a, 2012).

## Trauma therapists' experiences of traumatization within the context of the workplace

Trauma therapists risk becoming secondarily and vicariously traumatized in their work with survivors of trauma due to the nature of traumatic work itself, which has been described as 'a contagion' if entered into without sufficient preparation and training (Herman, 1992). The lack of adequate time and resources such as clinical supervision for reflection can result in trauma and stress which can impact both upon the client and therapist (Canfield, 2005; Cunningham, 2003). In the New Zealand context, research studies have suggested that what is defined as 'stressful' includes the experience of direct traumatization through intimidation and direct violence by co-workers as well as oppressive systems of management (Beddoe et al., 1999; van Heugten, 1999). For example, workers involved in child abuse and protection face intense media scrutiny when their best efforts fail to bring a positive outcome and tragically a child dies. Reports related to the death of 'Baby P' in the United Kingdom identified systemic failures, including a lack of training and supervision of the workers involved and claims of 'harassment' within the investigating workers' employing organization (Fernandez and Allen, 2009). Such organizational factors are more widespread than ordinarily thought, with patterns of violence, rudeness and bullying evidenced by research studies (van Heugten, 1999, 2011). As my narrative within mental health services with Freda illustrated, sometimes these organizational factors are more prevalent when auditing regimes are introduced, when workers are asked to account for their time and have a limited number of sessions available for use. The focus on outcomes within tight time frames can make narratives of failure systemically based and inevitable (Pack, 2008).

As a consequence of these factors, many trauma therapists are reporting increasing disillusionment with the workplace and team as a safe place in which to practise and are entering into private practice or contracted work in an effort to gain greater control over how they work with clients and manage their day-to-day functioning (van Heugten, 1999, 2011). When organizations and teams focus on the individual client and ignore the wider sociopolitical context in which trauma and abuse occur, this residual focus tends to conflict with trauma therapists' personal philosophies, theory and practice (Pack, 2004). If unaddressed, the effects of working with trauma can have wide-ranging implications for the organization as a whole. Individual experiences of vicarious traumatization can have a destabilizing effect on the teams in which workers are vicariously traumatized, which in turn can have a ripple effect on organizational functioning (Johnson and Hunter, 1997; Pack, 2004, 2010a, 2010b, 2010c; Sexton, 1999).

Adding to this movement into private practice is the increased interest in exposure to patterns of interaction known as workplace harassment and 'bullying'. Bullying is most often referred to as a pattern of behaviour or interaction usually by a manager higher up the organizational hierarchy towards a worker under their line management. A range of offensive behaviours are included in the definitions of bullying and harassment and there are common features reported. For example, there are often repeated patterns of interaction, where there are humiliating and denigrating comments made about a worker by another in the workplace, and a lack of information is given or fully discussed to enable the employee to fulfil work tasks and responsibilities in an informed way. There can be marginalizing of the voice and contribution of the worker within the team effort leading to isolation of the worker which keeps the cycle of abuse and humiliation going. For example, managers may be said to bully or harass by a deliberate exclusion of the victim from teamwork by a lack of invitation to meetings and being kept involved in project updates, leading to a loss of confidence and withdrawal by the victim (van Heugten, 2011). In the counsellor-participants study, they expressed views of feeling constrained by the reporting requirements that were sensitive to changes within the organization that contracted them to provide trauma therapy to claimants (Pack, 2004). In this sense, the problems were more systemic than being deliberately individual and personally based. These issues in the workplace were triggered by both the nature of the work, and by the counsellor-participants' 'survivor status' as they were living through their engagement with trauma in a primary sense (as having lived through personal experiences of trauma) and in a vicarious sense (witnessing the trauma of their clients). Third, the reporting requirements disadvantaged the client and counsellor in a way that was seen as a third form of abuse. The organizational abuse in the third example compounded the vicarious traumatization that was a routine feature of working with trauma and trauma survivors' narratives.

## The counsellor-participants' views of how to maintain effectiveness in the workplace

Analysis of the interviews with the counsellor-participants illustrated that they developed strategies for understanding their clients' trauma by reflecting on their own healing from traumatic events and their experiences in working with their clients (Pack, 2004). This experiential knowledge developed throughout their careers (spanning between five and 30 years) through both their own personal and professional experiences. These integrated insights were drawn on to guide the therapeutic process and assist in the counsellor-participants' own resilience in maintaining their on-the-job effectiveness. This awareness enabled the counsellor-participants to continue to practise with sexually abused clients which by its nature includes working with disclosures that are deemed 'hard to hear', including accounts of incest, intergenerational patterns of abuse, suicide and self-harm (Pack, 2010a, 2010b).

The counsellor-participants further reported feeling a lack of security about finding ongoing sources of funding for therapy (Pack, 2012). Many of the counsellor-participants reported moving into private practice or group practices for a variety of reasons mirroring van Heugten's (1999) findings. For some, this movement was seen as a way of resolving conflicts with agency politics and protocols. Group practices were seen as helpful to developing a shared ethos of the work and to tailoring the workplace administratively to suit those working together. In both instances having greater control over the way the workplace was organized was considered important (Pack, 2012).

## The early years: was vicarious traumatization an issue?

What the counsellor-participants did refer to as 'traumatizing' was often related to the range of assessment/investigative and therapeutic roles that were required by various agencies in which they worked. These mixed roles were seen as conflicting with counsellors' efforts in therapy and their desire to assist clients to make positive change in their lives.

The demands of being in a dual role were discussed in relation to those counsellor-participants who worked within, for example, the justice and child protection systems. Sally discussed ethical dilemmas surrounding what was seen as sexual abuse under law and policy, both of which determined who was eligible for publicly funded therapy. These criteria effectively defined whom she could assist, which created an ethical dilemma related to continuing therapy when the client was unable to pay privately.

For Angela, writing assessments on behalf of clients for the funding of their therapy was traumatizing. It seemed that the writing of these reports did not fit with the approaches she had adopted in her work as a psychotherapist with psychodrama training or as a more active collaborator:

> Angela: Not all of them [full assessment and treatment plans] are as bad, but when they're really terrible, when it's really crushing, it can't help but affect your spirit, your whole spirit, even working with someone who is telling you these things. It's like your heart just punctures really. And it is quite hard to let go, that's why I think anyone working with only this work, it's pretty dangerous, I reckon. The risk of either being in it; that this world, your having to, sort of, make it smaller in a way to be able to survive yourself.

## The development of personal philosophies

The counsellor-participants discussed the evolution in their thinking about sexual abuse. An understanding of the structural reasons for inequality and oppression and the misuse of power in society became integrated insights that the counsellor-participants drew upon in their practice. While earlier in their career trauma may have been more of a sub-field of professional specialization, more latterly sexual abuse was described on a continuum of other traumas and oppressions. Therapeutically, the counsellor-participants viewed sexual abuse as being part of the wider context of other oppressions, many of which have their origins in society. Kevin referred to specific theorists to explain and rationalize his views and emphasize 'trauma' rather than 'sexual abuse' in his work:

> Kevin: Well, coming at it from a much broader perspective, I think that my work with trauma goes far beyond sexual abuse. I mean half my clients at the moment are physical trauma – direct physical trauma – some head injuries, some attacked with a razor, that kind of thing. So it's a broader kind of thing. So I see sexual abuse, I suppose, as a trauma among others and I think it is really important to highlight that. I suppose I feel quite strongly that it [sexual abuse] is not to be put into a special place. The reactions that people show are the same as what a war veteran has, that kind of thing. So I see it as putting it in that sense. I see sexual abuse in terms of my knowledge; philosophically the person is affected in every dimension. In the last two years, I've moved. I've worked for the last 10–14 years but for the last two to three years I've moved an enormous amount particularly in terms of my understanding. This is more based on van der Kolk [see for instance van der Kolk *et al.*, 1996], that we are processing it [trauma] in an entirely different part of our brain: it's not a rational experience it's a very primitive emotive, pre-verbal, kind of a reaction; and consequently a lot of therapeutic intervention needs to involve a point of view that doesn't try to rationalize it away, which was really what the first ten years of my work was doing.

The intergenerational patterns of abuse that the counsellor-participants daily witnessed, suggested that societal factors were among the reasons as to why sexual abuse occurs. Theorists who combine this kind of social/political or structural analysis within their theories were among those that the counsellor-participants found the most useful to draw upon in their work. To acknowledge the historical and cultural origins of abuse and oppression in society, and to avoid making similar assumptions, the counsellor-participants sought an analysis of the sociocultural and historical/political factors. Through her work with her clients, Kahlia had developed her own theory about a loosening of social mores in which sexual abuse occurred in post-colonized New Zealand:

> Kahlia: I think New Zealand in particular is very bad in terms of the prevalence of sexual abuse, and my theory would be, like, I can't remember who it is wrote stuff about how come people left so long ago to come here from so far away; and being so far away, they weren't so accountable to society. So the boundaries are lost and then, of course, it [sexual abuse] becomes intergenerational and happens because people don't do their own personal work. Why it [sexual abuse] originally happens. I don't know. I think sexuality and the power and control issues around it [sexual abuse] are huge and I think New Zealand in particular has a long history of, you know, all that happens here or has happened in the past. I've been sexually abused. It wasn't an issue, well of course, it naturally had many consequences, but it wasn't confronted for many years. But it

just totally wipes people and their lives and the consequences of what they decide the world's about and why it happens [sexual abuse]. It is so important for people to get an opportunity to really explore their beliefs and cultures and values.

Drawing from an eclectic range of theories was considered 'useful' by counsellor-participants. Sally found a rationale for her practice in the writings of the 'new trauma therapy', epitomized by the foundational work of Herman (1992) and Briere (1996). In a similar way to these theorists, she refers to the power inequalities that exist across history, generations, socio-economic classes and cultures as being associated with her understanding of abuse and oppression and the need for social education for prevention:

> Sally: I think it is a mixture of theories and certainly I've found people like John Briere's [1996] model, really useful and Judith Herman's [1992] really useful. And it's interesting: it's often those people who we've heard talk at conferences and then you read more about their theories. I'm not a psychoanalytical person so I don't follow that theory. It doesn't appeal to me …

> I think they [Herman (1992) and Briere (1996)] fit in well without dragging out the theoretical model. My own belief is that abuse is something that is perpetuated from generation to generation so if one can do some really early childhood education that prevents this, that long term, and you're probably talking a generation or so, there would be much less abuse. Because abuse is not a new thing it has been going on for generations and I think back to historical readings of Victorian times when there was a very high level of abuse and it was because it was really about oppression and having power over somebody. And in Victorian times, the lord of the manor could do what he liked to his servants. Class was a factor then. I don't believe that class is a factor any longer, particularly not in New Zealand. I believe it's much more of a learned behaviour. It's not inherent in us. If we were abused we are more likely to abuse.

## Promoting anti-oppressive practice within organizations

The counsellor-participants' narratives suggested that an anti-oppressive approach is helpful in the field of sexual abuse and trauma counselling work. Ideally this philosophy is acknowledged by the organizations employing practitioners working in this arena (Pack, 2012). However, counsellor-participants suggested that for some organizations, emancipatory strengths-based practices may only be possible if their philosophies are better aligned with the philosophies of the professionals involved. This in turn would require training and supervising staff to encourage a shared vision, set of values, frame of reference and mandate for working together. Service users need to be reconceptualized as collaborators to become part of the multidisciplinary team in this re-visioning process. Effective teamwork, as Opie (2000) discovered in her research on multidisciplinary teams, occurs when there is a shared vision held by team members, an organizational discourse of success, a flattened organizational structure and knowledge about each profession represented on the multidisciplinary team.

## Challenging narratives of shame and disbelief

The counsellor-participants suggested that agencies engaged in trauma therapy need to find ways of challenging their own discourses that tend to doubt, disbelieve and objectify the narratives of survivors and those narratives of survival communicated via the counsellors and other treatment providers who care for them. The client's view of the situation, or the meanings attributed to events by the client, are the focus of the assessment within strengths-based social work, and this definition of 'assessment' offers an alternative paradigm for reporting (Saleeby, 1997: 63–4) that is closer to the modes in which counsellor-participants say that they work. The use of classificatory systems, such as the DSM, represents the language and frame of reference of the expert following models of individual pathology. However, the client's experience within strengths-based approaches is the mandated frame of reference for working. The client's view of the world is trustworthy and needs to be affirmed together with the opinion of the counsellor or treatment provider involved in providing care.

## The implications for practice

Emancipatory and strengths-based approaches challenge discourses of disbelief that surround trauma work by endorsing what people say. The theoretical approaches the counsellor-participants described as informing their work with trauma survivors assisted them to both understand and assist their clients, and they ameliorated the impact of vicarious traumatization. The organizations themselves were connected to the experience of vicarious traumatization when the reporting requirements and roles did not align to the ways in which the counsellor-participants worked.

Using emancipatory and strengths-based approaches within the field of trauma recovery may require interventions beyond individual therapy, involving political action, advocacy, systemic approaches, for example coordination of the professionals already involved and working for wider social change. For instance, a strengths-based, anti-oppressive assessment could more rigorously utilize the resources identified during assessment which might include resources found in local communities, families or *whanau* (*whanau* is a Māori term for extended family), as well as those used by professionals. This perspective challenges the role of the expert professional and re-conceptualizes the helping relationship. This challenges the idea that the therapist represents the means of all healing and rather articulates the therapist as a facilitator of the process with a role in identifying, coordinating and supporting the client's own efforts towards healing.

Trauma therapists, whose training is based in formulating and assessing in more traditional frameworks, may find strengths-based approaches challenging to their own sense of professionalism. Some may consider their professionalism compromised by adopting such approaches, which use different frames from the traditional diagnosis-and-cure formula of the medical model.

Adopting such an approach would require a new framework and new vision for some agencies but, through this process, the evolution of new monitoring, feedback and evaluation forms would ensure a narrowing of the gap that now exists between theory or agency requirements and the counsellors' frameworks for practice.

Working from a position of strength, rather than deficit, has many implications for how trauma therapists work with their clients. Instead of requiring therapists to sift through details of the original trauma, a strengths-based approach may be more suitable protection for both the client and the therapist. This may challenge current funding guidelines that require details of the original abuse in the first few sessions in order to procure funding.

Assessment and goal-setting are an integral part of the healing process, especially when undertaken within a strengths-based approach.

The relationship between the funder, trauma therapist and client needs to be reformulated as colleagues involved in a collective 'therapeutic conversation' in which each takes responsibility for key roles to facilitate healing. Case management when working alongside trauma therapists could also be reformulated into adopting an emancipatory, strengths-based assessment process in developing case management plans with claimants more collaboratively.

Other ways in which organizations proactively work to support trauma therapists include the provision of quality clinical supervision that shares a range of characteristics described in the previous chapter. Assessing caseload balance (trauma versus non-trauma work) is also much recommended to both ameliorate the potential for vicarious traumatization and to assist in the process of rebounding from it (Saakvitne *et al.*, 1996). Providing education to prospective employees about the inevitable risks of engaging in the work of witnessing trauma disclosures daily needs to be frankly discussed by employers at the initial interviewing for staff. Full induction of new therapists in post is also crucial to staff retention and well-being. Professional development, education and training opportunities are needed as a feature that is embedded in the organization as a regular and ongoing strategy to support those who work in the field of trauma. A variety of theoretical approaches is needed as an essential 'toolkit' for the work of trauma therapists.

Lastly, an area we will turn to again in the next chapter is the provision of a comprehensive programme of employee supports including a well-designed and easily accessed CISM programme is another essential ingredient of trauma therapist well-being in an organizational context that we will explore in the next chapter as it has a well-developed evidence base of its own.

## Reflective questions

In each of these areas, managers and employers have responsibilities to attend to the ongoing needs of those therapists and other helping professionals who engage with trauma and trauma disclosures on a regular and frequent basis.

Consider the following areas in your own employment/organizational context and ask if there is insufficient provision of professional development and resources in your workplace.

If you belong to a professional association, union or network who can add strength to your voice, then that network or group may be part of your advocacy plan so that you avoid the position of being a lone voice in the wilderness. Here are some issues to reflect and discuss with colleagues:

- What are the specific needs of trauma therapists in your work/organizational/team practice context?
- What is a realistic and reasonable caseload when dealing with trauma disclosures?
- What is the best caseload mix (balancing practice activities and interests with other commitments such as research, teaching and policy)? Take a moment to consider your own ideal mix of activities in your work day.
- If your work mix of activities and interests is not ideally the way you want it, what needs to change or be adjusted?

- What are your three 'next steps' to obtaining the resources you need in the organization/private practice?
- Is there a role for networking with other trauma therapists to advocate and facilitate greater access to professional development and support options in your workplace/profession?
- Is social media helpful in finding and connecting with like-minded others, for example, connecting with colleagues on LinkedIn, Facebook or Twitter?
- How will you make your own self-care a priority in the workplace while balancing the needs of your clients and colleagues?

Now, let's turn back to summarize some of the counsellor-participants' key ideas in each of the areas just reflected upon (caseload balance, dealing with one's own survivor issues as a trauma therapist, meeting professional development needs).

### Balancing caseloads and practice interests

One of the key insights from the counsellor-participants involved in the research was that it was inherently unhealthy to focus exclusively on trauma and sexual abuse counselling to the exclusion of all other roles and work. One suggestion was that the agencies contracting for sexual abuse work take more active responsibility for limiting the number of cases that their treatment providers take on for abuse and trauma counselling (Johnson and Hunter, 1997).

The focus group guiding my research recommended that a maximum number of five sexual abuse cases should be on a trauma therapist's caseload at any one time. Clinical supervisors could also balance caseloads and interests more collaboratively. Clinical supervisors are in the best position to assess the impact of the work on the individual worker and the degree of vicarious traumatization present at any one time.

Achieving balance is more challenging for agencies who exclusively focus on trauma, domestic violence and abuse, and consequently these agencies need to develop protocols for addressing health and safety issues such as vicarious traumatization as an organizational priority.

Professional associations could also support these principles by including them within their ethical guidelines and professional expectations and educational and training goals related to the potential for the vicarious traumatization among its professional members. Raising awareness within training courses and regular meetings may alert members of the signposts to becoming vicariously traumatized so that they can take ameliorative action.

Alongside this education, there needs to be active mentoring of less experienced therapists with those who have been working for five or more years in the field of trauma. The purpose of such mentoring would be to provide positive role models for younger staff members from whom they could learn some of the themes of resiliency that were evident among the counsellor-participants interviewed for this research (Pack, 2004, 2012).

### *Organizations employing workers who deal with survivors of sexual assault*

There are health and safety issues that need to be routinely addressed within organizations working with traumatic disclosures. The risks of engaging potentially traumatic material need to be explicit during recruitment. This research suggests that the risks can be ameliorated if there is sufficient support for workers to draw from a range of theoretical frameworks in an organization that models collegial behaviour and relationships.

Literature suggesting the possible cumulative effects of continued contact with traumatic material from clients needs to be honestly and frankly raised with job applicants and prospective employees. Training courses and practicum placements need also to alert entering students to the potential risks to their psychological health of their involvement in trauma-related helping. Alongside the vicarious traumatization literature, literature suggesting more positive outcomes needs also to be made available to provide a balance of perspectives from which individuals can select. A range of responses can then inform trauma therapists' views about the work they are undertaking. An established trauma therapist may be able to mentor or buddy a new worker and assist in educating them on a range of responses they have had in working with traumatic material.

### *Meeting the ongoing needs of workers*

Once employed, opportunities to share experiences arising from the work in the trauma field, including information/education about vicarious traumatization, needs to be made available to new employees. For example, individual supervision may occur alongside peer networks or groups; training workshops on anti-oppressive practice, as a means of ameliorating vicarious traumatization could be provided with employer support. Critical-reflective modes of reviewing one's practice as a means of debriefing workers from trauma would seem helpful to ameliorating the impact of the work (Fook, 1996; Fook *et al.*, 2000; Napier and Fook, 2001). Information on worker rights through access to union representatives, may assist in supporting workers to collectively advocate for conditions of employment that support their work. It is important that these areas of support and training are not superimposed with performance appraisal (Pack, 2012).

### *The needs of survivor therapists*

Personal therapy needs to be available to workers who find that there are issues of their own abuse or trauma intruding into their day-to-day work. Personal therapy is one of the means by which workers encountering triggers to their own experience of abuse and oppression may use therapy to feedback insights and ways of being into their own emerging theories of practice. Critical-reflective practice in which trauma therapists can engage in an ongoing analysis of themes in their work would seem helpful in tandem with personal therapy (Fook *et al.*, 2000; Napier and Fook, 2001). Therefore, the linkages between personal therapy of the trauma therapist as a model for informing their practice needs to be affirmed by employers and contracting organizations. In the past, survivor therapists have been criticized for lacking objectivity to undertake the work and were asked by their funding agency to leave the field for the duration of their personal therapy. While this may be helpful for some therapists, the research with the counsellor-participants suggests that survivor therapists, who undertake their own therapy, develop resources and insight that, over time, become a valuable basis for their practice (Pack, 2012).

## The future

In looking towards the future, research with the counsellor-participants suggests that there are ways in which trauma therapists can be supported by their teams and employing organizations to remain effective on the job. Therapists need to be proactively encouraged and educated to develop an awareness of vicarious traumatization in their daily lives and work. Building on earlier chapters, the findings of previous research also underlines the importance of trauma therapists sampling and integrating into their practice a wide range of theoretical approaches (Pack, 2010a, 2010b). These approaches, which include narrative, strengths-based and emancipatory frameworks, provide a way for workers to connect with themselves, which naturally fosters effective connections with clients, colleagues and their significant others. Frameworks that integrate the various strands of these theories – including trauma-informed theories of practice – the counsellor-participants found to be the most relevant. Within trauma-informed theory the therapeutic relationship creates the climate in which clients can re-discover their own innate resilience and, through this awareness, be enabled to carry this knowledge into action in their everyday lives. The findings of my research suggest that there needs to be a realignment in the philosophies of the funding organizations involved in trauma therapy towards an approach consistent with these aims and with the practice of the therapists.

Maintaining relationship is the primary theme of this research which protects the trauma therapist from the fragmenting sense of disjuncture that is a key experience of the work. Thus conceptualized, prevention strategies include trauma therapists being firmly grounded in theoretical frameworks that provide a context for establishing and maintaining connection on a variety of levels: with the self, with others including clients, with their employing organizations and with the wider social discourses in which their work is located (Pack, 2012).

Employers, professional associations, training establishments and contracting agencies have responsibilities to alert trauma therapists to the potential impact of continued work in the field of trauma. Literature discussing the protective factors that build resiliency in dealing with traumatic disclosures should be available to staff, alongside the literature cautioning their continued engagement in trauma-related therapy. This would provide a more balanced picture of the potential long-term impact of work in the field of trauma on individual therapists. Second, trauma therapists require continuing opportunities and encouragement to share experience of their practice, including experiences of vicarious traumatization and burnout/compassion fatigue to provide a critical-reflective space in which to re-author their personal narratives and to evolve and develop theories of practice over time. Programmes of continuing professional development need to prioritize such goals.

## Resources on dealing with bullying and harassment in the workplace

If you are experiencing bullying or harassment in the workplace, the following websites and resouces offer information, support and advocacy:

*Bully Zero Australia Foundation*

> Includes a section on bullying in the workplace and how to respond as well as contact via email and freephone:

> http://bzaf.org.au

*Fairwork Ombudsman Australia*

This weblink provides free advice for employees focusing on employee rights, entitlements and agreements and awards in Australia. Definitions of bullying and harassment and resources are included:

www.fairwork.gov.au

*Anti-discrimination Commission (Australia)*

The Commission leads the promotion and protection of all human rights in Australia, including employee rights with independent advice for employees. Publications and weblinks to other resources are available:

www.humanrights.gov.au

*The Workplace Bullying Institute*

An American website offering useful resources about workplace bullying, including definitions and advice about what to do in different scenarios and contexts:

www.workplacebullying.org

*ReachOut.com*

A website focusing on workplace bullying, abuse and violence in Australia:

http://au.reachout.com/Tough-Times/Bullying-Abuse-and-Violence/Bullying?gclid =Cj0KEQjw9o-vBRCO0OLi2PfPkI8BEiQA8pdF4AbTTw0yoAJIBBgeENCzOwQ9ZCs5ijqkru NSO3qq9dwaAr768P8HAQ

*Worksafe New Zealand*

Guidelines developed in New Zealand for managing workplace bullying released in February 2014 including several self-assessment and self-help tools:

www.business.govt.nz/worksafe/news/releases/2014/worksafe-new-zealand-releases-guidelines-for-managing-workplace-bullying

## Further reading if you are considering a move into private practice as a trauma therapist

van Heugten, K. (1999). Social workers who move into private practice: A study of the issues that arise for them (unpublished doctoral dissertation). University of Canterbury, Christchurch, New Zealand.

van Heugten, K. (2011). *Social work under pressure: How to overcome stress, fatigue and burnout in the workplace*. London: Jessica Kingsley.

## References

Beddoe, L., Appleton, C. and Maher, B. (1999). Social workers and violence. *Social Work Now, 12* (April), 36–42.

Briere, J. (1996). *Therapy for adults molested as children: Beyond survival.* New York: Springer.

Canfield, J. (2005). Secondary traumatisation, burnout, and vicarious traumatisation: A review of the literature as it relates to therapists who treat trauma. *Smith College Studies in Social Work, 75* (2), 81–102.

Chouliara, Z., Hutchison, C. and Karatzias, T. (2009). Vicarious traumatisation in practitioners who work with adult survivors of sexual violence and child sexual abuse: Literature review and directions for future research. *Counselling and Psychotherapy Research: Linking Research with Practice, 9* (1), 47–56.

Cunningham, M. (2003). Impact of trauma work on social work clinicians: Empirical findings. *Social Work*, *48* (4), 451–9.

Fernandez, C. and Allen, V. (2009). Baby Peter: Now his father bids to cash in with a demand for £200,000 compensation. *Mail Online*. 12 August. Retrieved from: www.dailymail.co.uk/news/article-1205888/Baby-P-Now-father-bids-cash-demand-200-000-compensation.html (accessed 2 March 2016).

Fook, J. (1996). *The reflective researcher: Social workers' theories of practice research.* St Leonards, NSW: Allen & Unwin.

Fook, J., Ryan, M. and Hawkins, L. (2000). *Professional expertise: Practice, theory and education for working with uncertainty.* London: Whiting & Birch.

Herman, J. (1992). *Trauma and recovery.* New York: Basic Books.

Johnson, C. N. E. and Hunter, M. (1997). Vicarious traumatisation in counsellors working in the New South Wales assault service: An exploratory study. *Work and Stress*, *11* (4), 319–28.

Napier, L. and Fook, J. (Eds). (2001). *Breakthroughs in practice: Theorising critical moments in social work.* London: Whiting & Birch.

Opie, A. (2000). *Thinking teams/thinking clients: Knowledge-based teamwork.* New York: Columbia University Press.

Pack, M. J. (2004). Sexual abuse counsellors' responses to stress and trauma: A social work perspective. *Social Work Review: Journal of New Zealand Association of Social Workers*, *16* (1), 19–25.

Pack, M. (2008). The concept of hope in gestalt therapy: It's usefulness for ameliorating vicarious traumatisation. *Gestalt Australia and New Zealand Journal*, *3* (2), 59–71.

Pack, M. J. (2010a). Revisions to the therapeutic relationship: A qualitative inquiry into sexual abuse therapists' theories for practice as a mitigating factor in vicarious traumatisation. *Social Work Review: Journal of New Zealand Association of Social Workers*, *12* (1), 73–82.

Pack, M. J. (2010b). Discovering an integrated framework for practice: A qualitative investigation of theories used by social workers working as sexual abuse therapists. *Journal of Social Work Practice*, *25* (1), 79–93.

Pack, M. J. (2010c). Career themes in the lives of sexual abuse counsellors: A qualitative inquiry into therapist responses to stress and trauma. *New Zealand Journal of Counselling*, *30* (2), 75–92.

Pack, M. (2012). Vicarious traumatisation: An organisational perspective. *Social Work Now: The Practice Journal of Child, Youth and Family*, *50*, 14–23.

Rabu, M., Moltu, C., Binder, P. and McLeod, J. (2015). How does practising psychotherapy affect the personal life of the therapist? A qualitative inquiry of senior therapists' experiences. *Psychotherapy Research*. doi: 10.1080/10503307.2015.1065354

Saakvitne, K. W., Pearlman, L. A. and the staff of the Traumatic Stress Institute (1996). *Transforming the pain: A workbook on vicarious traumatization.* New York: Norton.

Saleebey, D. (Ed.). (1997). *The strengths perspective in social work practice* (2nd edn). New York: Longman.

Sexton, L. (1999). Vicarious traumatisation of counsellors and effects on their workplaces. *Journal of Guidance and Counselling*, *27* (3), 393–404.

van der Kolk, B., McFarlane, A. C. and Weisaeth, L. (Eds). (1996). *Traumatic stress: The effects of overwhelming experience on mind, body, and society.* New York: Guildford Press.

van Heugten, K. (1999). Social workers who move into private practice: A study of the issues that arise for them (unpublished doctoral dissertation). University of Canterbury, Christchurch, New Zealand.

van Heugten, K. (2011). *Social work under pressure: How to overcome stress, fatigue and burnout in the workplace.* London: Jessica Kingsley.

# Chapter 7    **Critical incident stress management**

## Self-care in the workplace

I think again of that prison case when I worked with this person and the father abused her more than once and she really had made enormous progress. She went out the weekend before she was released and she was once again abused by her father. When she was released she hanged herself because she couldn't see her way out. She was about twenty-six at that stage but the incest happened yet again. So that was a tragedy. I sought critical incident debriefing. My reaction at the time and even now – it [debriefing] changed my belief in suicide, very dramatically, because I realized the client made the very best choice she saw possible at the time.

*Sally, counsellor-participant discussing the most difficult case she had encountered as a trauma therapist and her thoughts about how critical incident stress debriefing (CISD) assisted her to develop reframed understandings of the tragic and disturbing events involving her client*

### Introduction

This chapter describes the debates in the research literature surrounding the provision of CISM and outlines the implications for trauma therapists' experience of vicarious traumatization. As discussed in the previous chapter, employers have a moral and ethical as well as legal responsibility to ensure the safety of workers within their contracting organization. As part of a self-care strategy, therefore, trauma therapists need to ensure that they have knowledge of what is best practice in CISM programmes so that they know whether they need to explore other practice contexts, workplaces and, for private practitioners, contracting environments that better support their needs.

The literature reviewed suggests that CISD as an intervention needs to be offered as part of a comprehensive programme of CISM that is integrated and sensitive to the organizational context (Pack, 2013). Strengths-based principles need to underpin an integrated CISM policy that is sensitive to differences in individual responses, organizational contexts and diverse fields of trauma therapy practice. Adaptations of Mitchell's (1983) original model of CISM, which aims at mitigating the potential negative impact of critical incidents encountered in the workplace while enhancing personal resilience, are discussed with reference to recent critiques of this model.

### Background

The counsellor-participants encountered events from which they valued a range of CISM services, including CISM debriefing. Mostly their CISD occurred within an established relationship in clinical supervision (Pack, 2009). Whether CISM is essential to therapist and helper self-care is, however, a contested field. The debates in the research literature surrounding the provision of psychological debriefing following critical events are many and varied. They include queries about which approaches and interventions should be used and what constitutes 'best practice'. CISM literature falls into a number of categories – evaluations of existing frameworks, their applications in differing contexts and reviews on the basis of personal experience, opinion and commentary (Lewis, 2003). Lewis further asserts that most literature on the subject of psychological debriefing consists of commentary stimulating debate within the field. Within this commentary three strands of opinion are evident: 'Proponents of the intervention, critics of the intervention, and personal "war stories" with no empirical data' (Lewis, 2003: 331).

To explore the models that were useful to therapists in their work, I embarked upon a systematic literature review (Pack, 2013) and undertook research on the subject with mental health and child protection social workers (Pack, 2014b) to explore the themes identified earlier with the counsellor-participants (Pack, 2009). The purpose of the literature review framing this chapter is to chart some of the major themes in the argument for and against psychological debriefing, in the hope of stimulating further reflection for trauma therapists on the usefulness of various models of CISM to maintaining their self-care. Second, the intention of presenting a systemic review of previous literature on CISM is to clarify the positioning of trauma therapy within these debates, to create new definitions in the process of critical reflection (Pack, 2013).

The literature on CISM is multidisciplinary with nursing, fire services, police, emergency work, trauma therapy and allied health professions contributing to the commentary about CISM models and their value to practice and practitioners. The term 'psychological debriefing' is an umbrella term that covers a range of interventions. These interventions are typically short-term and aimed at alleviating long-term distress and preventing the development of PTSD (Devilly *et al.*, 2006). CISD and defusing are specific approaches offered within the more generic term of 'psychological debriefing'. These concepts are given different emphasis in some CISM models or the more recent notion of 'psychological first aid'.

## Search strategy

A search was run in the databases Cinahl, PubMed, Social Services Abstracts, PsychInfo and SSCI using the keywords: 'critical incident stress' and 'trauma therap*' (the * is used in a format for electronic database searching to expand options and to increase possible 'hits' so enhancing the chances of finding a more complete literature to be reviewed). A second broader search was also tried using the keywords: 'critical incident stress'. Publications were selected within the past ten years to show recent developments in the field of CISM since Mitchell and Everly's model of CISM developed from the late 1980s and was refined and elaborated throughout the 1990s and beyond. Seminal works in the field that were cited in the recent literature were then followed up to put the commentary and debates into their historical context. Those papers that were cited from the context of critical incidents encountered in the helping services were selected, as I discovered there was a broader literature about survivor narratives to a variety of disasters that were unrelated to the helping professions directly, so these articles were less relevant to the focus of this paper (Pack, 2013).

Systematic reviews and meta-analyses were less frequently encountered, therefore, qualitative or mixed method evaluations were included alongside personal commentary that added to the debates about the efficacy of CISM and specific interventions within these models. The 'personal war stories', 'proponents' and 'critics' of CISD earlier mentioned by Lewis (2003: 331) were all sought to show the range, depth and breadth of debate in the literature as it relates to the helping professions and in particular to trauma therapy. Selection of articles was made on the basis of titles involving these search terms, using Lewis's debate typology of 'proponents' and 'critics' of CISM as the criteria for inclusion. Commentaries and 'personal war stories' were read as background to the main evaluations and systematic reviews of recent research. Articles written in English or available with an English translation were included as the author's language was English.

Content analysis was undertaken and the results were analysed thematically. Once the articles were read and the content of each article analysed, each article was categorized as being primarily for, against or undecided in relation to the debate about the efficacy and effectiveness of CISM and related interventions. This analysis positioned each research article within the current debates in the literature about CISM. The majority of research publications reviewed were either supportive of existing models or gave an undecided view of the efficacy and effectiveness of CISM. Difficulties were identified in the majority of substantive studies reviewed, in conceptually defining CISM and related terminology, and due to methodological shortcomings of existing evaluative studies in the field (Pack, 2013).

## Background

CISM has been described as a 'comprehensive, multi-component, well integrated work-based programme that is designed to assist emergency service workers' (Robinson, 2000: 92). The elements of CISD within the CISD process include the detailed disclosure of facts, thoughts and emotional reactions, and sensory material linked to the event or incident. Coping factors under CISM programmes include education about traumatic stress, normalization of responses, anticipatory troubleshooting and planning for the future, and group support factors where a reassuring and supportive environment is facilitated by a peer or leader (Lewis, 2003).

Mitchell, who developed the original model of CISD, together with colleagues, counters critics' arguments that CISD was always seen as insufficient as a 'stand-alone' intervention by saying that as an intervention it was always envisaged by its authors to form part of a comprehensive, integrated approach or a part of CISM (Everly et al., 2001).

Historically, approaches to CISM developed originally from an identified need within the military during war time to debrief from events encountered by war veterans in the course of combat (Plaggemars, 2000). The thinking at that time was that group CISD as an intervention enables soldiers to return to the war zone by ameliorating 'shell shock' or PTSD. Other historical influences include the development of crisis intervention models, the growth in knowledge about recovery from trauma and the specialization of therapies within psychology (Robinson, 2000). Herman (1992) discusses the shame and disbelief that historically has surrounded trauma that was relaxed with the return of Vietnam War veterans and the feminist movement of the 1970s. From this era onwards, the rights of trauma survivors entered the public consciousness and their rights were acknowledged by the provision of appropriate services.

## Recent developments

More recently critics of CISM conclude that its primary intervention, CISD, does not prevent psychological conditions such as PTSD and, furthermore, may be harmful if used indiscriminately (Boudreaux and McCabe, 2000; Devilly and Cotton, 2003). Current thinking is that CISD facilitators should not push people to reveal anything that is still too upsetting for them to discuss, as this may cause additional harm by encouraging participants to re-experience the traumatic event at a time when healthy denial and avoidance may facilitate recovery (Devilly and Cotton, 2003). The argument for early intervention in CISM as a preventative model is that the provision of such programmes usually involves three distinct approaches. The first is waiting and screening those who are likely to need assistance; second, allowing natural social networks to operate to heal; and third, proactive early intervention (Dyregrov, 1997). Devilly and Cotton (2003) assert that waiting and assessing to target interventions such as CISD to those who are deemed to need the intervention is the ethical way forwards to applying the practice of psychological intervention following critical incidents.

## Definitions of CISM: key elements

Several theorists have been influential in setting the framework for CISM approaches around which the debates about the efficacy of CISM have emerged subsequently. These theorists include Mitchell, Everly and Flannery and their founding work in the American context. In the Australian context, Robinson's interpretations of CISD see the process integrated within a CISM programme in a less prescriptive, more holistic way. Robinson (2000, 2007) acknowledges that stress reactions invoked by a critical incident may vary significantly from person to person, determined by a range of factors, including the nature of the incident, personality characteristics, value and belief systems, prior experiences of trauma, and the quality of leadership and support systems in the organization (Robinson, 2000). In light of this, the process of debriefing requires a clear definition and structure that is able to be tailored to the individual as well as the work team. In this way a prescriptive, one-size-fits-all approach is considered detrimental to individual resilience as some individuals given the time and resources naturally 'bounce back' without any more formal intervention than spending quality time within emotionally sustaining relationships (Devilly and Cotton, 2004).

CISD as an intervention is considered best offered as part of a comprehensive programme of CISM that is integrated into the organization (Caine and Ter-Bagdasarian, 2003). Such a programme needs to involve the organization as a whole with teams and allied professionals rather than solely adopting an individual focus. However, although current evidence suggests that employers have a duty of care for employees in high-risk occupations such as helpers in the acute and emergency services, confusion abounds about the most appropriate forms of intervention (Pack, 2014a; Regel, 2007). Mitchell's (1983) model of CISM and later developments draw from crisis intervention that is deemed important when dealing with helping professionals. As professional helpers are likely to evolve and adapt their own coping resources following a critical incident, there is a brief time immediately after the event when workers are more open to processing their own responses to distressing material encountered on the job (Robinson, 2000). If this opportunity is missed by too long a wait between the incident and opportunity for those helping professionals to process what happened and their responses, this opportunity can be lost irretrievably (Robinson, 2000). Timing of intervention is, therefore, critical, which is an advantage of Mitchell *et al*.'s (2003) model of CISM and, within this overarching model, interventions such as CISD, offered on a team basis, ideally within 24–48 hours of the event (Donnelly and Siebert, 2009).

The organizational culture and context are thought to mediate responses to critical events (Devilly *et al.*, 2006). There is a growing body of research that asserts that at the organizational level employers who accord priority to workplace strategies to improve the morale of employees contribute to job satisfaction and resilience (Devilly *et al.*, 2006). For example, in critical care nursing, around one-half of all employee turnover is thought to be due to work stress, much of which is unacknowledged by the employing organization (Caine and Ter-Bagdasarian, 2003). Therefore, Mitchell *et al.*'s (2003) model of CISM has been adapted and applied to a variety of organizational contexts where staff are dealing with trauma and life-and-death issues on a daily basis in an effort to improve staff retention and morale (Devilly *et al.*, 2006; Lane, 1993). There is evidence that staff impacted by critical events manifest their distress in various ways. Those symptoms most frequently reported by hospital workers dealing with critical events such as death of a colleague through suicide include sleep disturbance and 'intrusive thoughts about the victim' (Plaggemars, 2000: 91). Cognitive reframing of such beliefs is part of the focus of the CISD as a carefully paced, multi-stage intervention.

However, though organizations increasingly offer various forms of psychological intervention, the cost often discourages organizations to offer a comprehensive CISM programme (Pack, 2014a). As a consequence, employee assistance programmes tend to be left with the task of assessing those employees who are worst affected or who are referred by management following a critical event (Plaggemars, 2000). Alternatives to CISD as an intervention include the pared-down option of 'defusing' and less formalized 'peer support'. Both of these interventions are cited as having their value in the research literature, as they tend to be more cost-effective when compared with a more formal team debriefing intervention. The distinctions between CISD and defusing are less clearly defined in the literature, however, leading to difficulties comparing interventions as the elements of each approach offered within CISM models differ considerably. Yet critics of Mitchell's claims to knowledge argue that 'it appears that anything involving intervention for distressed or victimized individuals could be considered critical incident stress debriefing as it is currently defined (or, rather, not defined)' (Devilly and Cotton, 2004: 36).

Lane (1993) and Lewis (2003) also write with an emphasis on coping strategies and resilience in relation to CISD/CISM which combine strengths-based theories with CISD/CISM. Strengths-based theories are prevalent in recent directions in trauma therapy theories of practice and so are referred to as informing trauma therapy theory building around emerging definitions of CISD/CISM (Tuckey, 2007).

## Critical events

Definitions of critical events vary widely in the articles reviewed. For example, from a therapy perspective Bell (1995: 37) defines critical events as 'traumatic events'. Citing Figley (1995) 'traumatic events' are defined as falling into the categories of 'natural disasters' such as earthquakes, 'accidental catastrophes' such as motor vehicle accidents and 'human-induced catastrophes' such as acts of interpersonal violence and abuse. Lane (1993) defines critical incidents as being related to situations of death and dying encountered by health-care professionals.

Devilly and Cotton (2003: 148) mention 'terminology slippage' referring to the generalizing of critical incidents to events that in their view are not traumatic, such as co-worker conflict in the workplace. In this way Devilly and Cotton (2003: 144) conclude that

> frequently and particularly in applied contexts, terms are being used without operational definitions and are often used interchangeably. This makes inspecting the evidence behind the claims a murky and very difficult task.

This 'murkiness' is evident in evaluations of workplace psychological debriefing in relation to 'critical incidents' such as restructuring and redundancy in the workplace. In one study reviewed, for example, psychological debriefing through employee assistance programmes was found to be effective in assisting employees to verbalize their issues and construct alternative meaning from experience following redundancy (Plaggemars, 2000). Whether organizational change and restructuring can be defined as a 'critical event' in the same sense as an unexpected death of a client or colleague by suicide, for example, remains problematic in the literature, however.

In the critical events described to me during interviews with the counsellor-participants, there was a recurring theme in the content of 'critical incidents'. All of the participants described working with clients who were suicidal or decided not to continue with therapy and subsequently carried through with a suicide plan successfully, evoking existential despair and a range of issues about being human (Pack, 2009). This critical incident(s) was a major milestone in the career of the counsellor-participant and, if successfully navigated with the right support and debriefing, was seen as an essential part of their personal and professional growth (Pack, 2014b). Rabu *et al*., (2015) similarly found in their research into the impact of practising as a psychotherapist that critical incidents involving clients who attempted suicide were a major event that affected the personal life of a therapist. Specifically there were feelings of responsibility and guilt in the form of persistent thoughts that they could have changed the outcome by doing more.

## Support for interventions within CISM models

The majority of outcome studies suggest that those workers who participate in CISM programmes find it a valuable experience and in particular those programmes that include a CISD (Tuckey, 2007). Those aspects that are positively commented upon following group psychological debriefing include the sharing of experiences that normalize common responses (Tuckey, 2007). Other positive outcomes that have been reported include a reduction in alcohol abuse which has been identified as a co-morbid factor linked to traumatization among many professions, including those who work with trauma such as therapists and military personnel (Deahl, 2000; Deahl, *et al*., 2001).

## Evaluations of CISD

Positive feedback about the process of group debriefings as an intervention within CISM programmes has been documented in a variety of different contexts involving a diversity of 'critical events'. For example, police officers involved in the Oklahoma bombing used group and individual interventions with clinicians specializing in law enforcement issues following the event (Horn, 2002). Horn (2002: 314) noted that a prior history of trauma may either 'sensitise' or 'immunise' officers to subsequent trauma depending on whether or not they had worked through the earlier trauma. Therefore, a range of interventions was needed to be available to officers on a voluntary basis. Services included residential workshops, one-to-one sessions, chaplaincy and EMDR therapy with positive feedback from participants. The success of the debriefing was considered to arise from using clinicians who were familiar with the context of police work and by offering an eclectic range of interventions that officers could select voluntarily from in a supportive workshop environment.

CISD, used with employees undergoing job restructuring where redundancy is the outcome, has been found to have meaning-generating outcomes for the participants (Plaggemars,

2000). Downsizing-based CISD groups not only engender mutual and peer support, they can facilitate a productive adaption to loss and change which may assist in the quest for another job or in transitioning into retirement (Plaggemars, 2000).

While some reviewers of meta-analyses find mixed results to the efficacy of CISD evaluations, they also find a number of secondary gains that participants are found to make through engagement with the debriefing (Mitchell *et al.*, 2003).These gains include individual benefits such as emotional ventilation, stress management and reassurance that the range of stress responses is normal to experience. Enhancement of the work group process, interagency cooperation, and screening and referral for additional services were other secondary positive goals identified (Mitchell *et al.*, 2003). One study of peer diffusers, for example, discovered that the involvement of peer diffusers in the workplace reduced lost employee time after critical incidents. Improved organizational culture and workplace health were noted as well as the peer diffusers' transferring enhanced skills to other work tasks (Freeman and Carson, 2006).

Similarly, the 'meaning-making' functions of group CISD have been discovered when workers discuss the suicide of clients and colleagues as critical events (Plaggemars, 2000). For example, a mental health nursing study in Northern Ireland found that CISD had good outcomes with a group of three research participants. All found the individual and group debriefing process validating of their experiences and offering hope for the future at the six-month follow-up (Irving and Long, 2001). The usefulness of combining group CISD with individual psychotherapy is mentioned as ideally forming part of a comprehensive programme of CISM (Galliano, 2002; Irving and Long, 2001). Induction of new employees with stress management education that encourages adaptive responses to events in the workplace is seen as important in dealing with critical incidents in a preventative sense (Lane, 1993; MacNab *et al.*, 2003).

Riddell and Clouse (2004) warn that critics who argue that CISD is at best ineffectual or at worse harmful may be throwing the baby out with the bathwater as they fail to understand that debriefing is part of a broader approach to the psychosocial needs of persons affected by trauma to promote resilience. Mitchell (2004) has entered the debate to point out that the majority of criticisms about CISD refer to what is a single session of debriefing that is not what the original model of CISM intended, as single-session debriefing would violate the guidelines of standards of CISM practice (Mitchell, 1983, Mitchell *et al.*, 2003).

## Critique

Critics of psychological debriefing assert that its meaning is problematic as the concept is defined in various ways. This lack of conceptual clarity leads to further difficulties of application and the scope of use across various contexts (Arendt and Elklit, 2001; Regel, 2007; Tuckey, 2007) and uniformity of process (Regel, 2007). The aims of use also lack definition, therefore, greater conceptual clarity is needed to determine if the evaluation of a diverse range of approaches and interventions actually refers to the CISD as an intervention and integrates with the more comprehensive term: CISM (van Emmerik *et al.*, 2002). Regel (2007) argues, for example, that the umbrella concept of 'psychological debriefing' and 'critical incident stress management' are widely used in the United Kingdom despite various misconceptions and misunderstandings about the terms. Some see CISM as an intervention as being the same as counselling, and these confusions in terminology reflect misunderstanding that is translated into multiple interpretations as to what is done in practice (Regel, 2007; van Emmerik *et al.*, 2002).

Therefore, given this lack of clarity of terminology and application, the criteria for the evaluation of the effectiveness of psychological debriefing also lack consensus in the literature (Lewis, 2003; MacNab *et al.*, 2003). One meta-analysis of 25 studies concludes four main criteria for success (Arendt and Elklit, 2001). These criteria include the definition of psychological debriefing's purpose which is to prevent psychological disorders such as the development of PTSD. However, there is a lack of consensus as to whether psychological debriefing and CISM have the same meaning (Devilly and Cotton, 2004). Second, there are queries as to whether the main intention of the umbrella term 'psychological debriefing' is primarily aimed at preventing PTSD (Regel, 2007).

More recently, the use of psychological debriefing is seen as a morale-boosting intervention, 'a gesture of employer support, rather than a clinical intervention influencing distress and clinical symptomatology' (Devilly and Cotton, 2004: 147). Other studies remain undecided about CISD's efficacy as there is still no consensus on whether single-session debriefing can contribute to the prevention of symptoms of chronic PTSD (van Emmerik *et al.*, 2002). The authors conclude in their meta-analysis of seven studies evaluating CISD as an intervention that: 'Critical incident stress debriefing has no efficacy in reducing symptoms of post-traumatic stress disorder and other trauma-related symptoms' (van Emmerik *et al.*, 2002: 769). Robertson *et al.*, (2004) concur with these authors and conclude that CISD may be at best neutral in its after-effects but for some may be harmful (van Emmerik *et al.*, 2002).

These findings are supported by evidence that single-session debriefing is generally considered less helpful by the participants (Devilly and Cotton, 2003; Robertson *et al.*, 2004; Tuckey, 2007). Devilly and Cotton (2003) argue that CISD as a one-off intervention may cause harm based on their review of randomized controlled trials. However, Robinson (2004) counters these criticisms by saying that Devilly and Cotton are operating on a number of common misunderstandings and a lack of evidence to support their assertions. CISD was never designed as a stand-alone intervention. Despite attempts for Mitchell to clarify the use of the terms CISM as the model and CISD as the intervention, throughout the 1990s, misunderstanding of these two concepts continues (Robinson, 2004).

There are problems reported with the randomized controlled trials reviewed by Devilly and Cotton (2003) which are considered to be methodologically flawed. For example, Robinson (2004) asserts that the studies chosen by Devilly and Cotton for review fail to acknowledge intervening variables throughout the study. The critical incident stress models are blamed for traumatizing citizens through unsolicited helping efforts by the public, for example, after 9/11. Further the assertion that psychological debriefing has created an industry for Robinson (2004: 31) 'paints a picture of exploitative, unethical behaviour that is unfounded'. Gist and Devilly (2002: 741) propose the way forward as a more structured, 'stepped' set of interventions that can be individually tailored, two-to-four weeks after the critical incident. This intervention would be offered on the assumption that brief cognitive therapy has efficacy in treating PTSD in those populations deemed to be 'high risk'. How 'high risk' is defined has yet to be elucidated, however.

Another randomized controlled trial of three levels of critical stress intervention among ambulance staff evaluated the effectiveness of three intervention strategies and attempted to correlate symptoms with the severity of incident and level of intervention (MacNab *et al.*, 2003). The authors discovered that requests for CISD among ambulance staff were uncommon which could be related to the reluctance of unionized staff to self refer to a co-ordinator who was unknown to them for debriefing. The other possible explanation for the lack of uptake of critical incident stress debriefing may be accounted by the lack of awareness of critical incident stress by the ambulance workers (MacNab *et al.*, 2003). The authors conclude that caution is needed when providing psychological debriefing due to the paucity of well-designed evaluations of CISD (MacNab *et al*, 2003).

## Methodological issues

Evaluations of psychological debriefing interventions have been reviewed by evidence-based researchers, revealing a number of methodological shortcomings of the existing studies (Everly *et al.*, 1999). These shortcomings involve the fact that sample sizes are often small, the studies are retrospective rather than prospective and there is an absence of control groups (Regel, 2007). The lack of uniformity of processes, timing variances in the delivery of specific interventions, low response rates and lack of generalizability across different contexts and traumatic events, confounds the evaluation of effectiveness (Everly *et al.*, 1999). Furthermore, there is limited evidence that interventions after traumatic events such as psychological debriefing have preventative effects in terms of preventing PTSD (Robertson *et al.*, 2004).

What exactly 'effectiveness' is seems difficult to define with the symptomatology of PTSD being the main outcome measure. Regel (2007) suggests that there is a gap in the research literature as there are no studies assessing the impact of other symptoms of traumatization which may involve other markers of social and occupational functioning such as alcohol and drug use. Robertson *et al.* (2004: 108) concur with this conclusion and call for 'a broader range of outcome measures' when researching the efficacy of CISD.

Despite the ongoing debate about definitions of CISM models and the phases of intervention encompassed within these approaches, there is an opinion that through academic debate, progress is being made in defining the key concepts and elements (Flannery and Everly, 2004; Suveg, 2007). The challenge according to Flannery and Everly (2004: 327) is for standardized definitions of 'critical events' and intervention protocols to be developed. Reliable outcome measures that are tested by formally trained personnel who are inducted in the standardized procedures are required (Flannery and Everly, 2004). While more rigorously conducted research using controlled experimental design is recommended, the ethical issue of withholding treatment to the control group is noted as a major obstacle in research using control groups (Devilly and Cotton, 2003; Flannery and Everly, 2004).

## The implications for trauma therapy

The findings from the studies reviewed have implications for trauma therapists as facilitators of CISM programmes, both for colleagues and with clients as part of clinical practice. Trauma therapy educators who prepare students for the many challenges they will face that are inherent in the practicum environment, and for qualified trauma therapists who encounter critical incidents on the job, CISM programmes can provide a range of options supporting professional effectiveness, well-being and staff retention.

Critical incident stress debriefers quote numerous examples illustrating the efficacy of the group process for participants (Lane, 1993; Morrison, 2007; Pritchard, 2004; Spitzer and Burke, 1993; Spitzer and Neely, 1993). Within organizations such as hospitals, trauma therapists are seen as ideally qualified and positioned to offer CISM programmes in their employing workplaces as they are used to collaborating with a variety of emergency helping professionals (Lane, 1993; Spitzer and Burke, 1993; Spitzer and Neely, 1993). A holistic view of people; a focus on social justice establishing rights and responsibilities for all; an ability to respect difference and think broadly, influencing social change; and group work skills are among those characteristics and competencies that make trauma therapists ideally suited to facilitate a range of critical incident stress interventions such as debriefing. Trauma therapy as a profession works on the margins of systems and with events that are routinely outside the usual range of human experience in contexts as diverse as child protection, health and welfare. In these contexts, the experience of working intensively with grief, loss and unexpected crises are an everyday feature of the work. Trauma therapists witness and work alongside their clients to support their resilience in the face of traumatic events. In a parallel way, trauma therapists are returning to consider the needs of their colleagues and of the workforce in relation to CISM.

The mental health stigma is avoided by CISD being conducted by multidisciplinary teams, including peers within the participants' own workplace (Pritchard, 2004). It is vital that the facilitators who conduct the process are well trained and have credibility in the eyes of the participants (Maher, 1999; Pritchard, 2004). The experience from those writing as critical incident stress debriefers is that being a trusted peer in the workplace fosters trust and flow in the group debriefing process (Lane, 1993; Maher, 1999; Pritchard, 2004). This view contrasts with some CISM policies, however, where independent support via employee assistance programmes is deemed more effective to target those most in need and likely to respond to formal CISD as an intervention (Devilly and Cotton, 2004). Confidentiality can be compromised with less formal models of debriefing involving peer supporters. Specifically untrained peer supporters without adequate training in CISD and strong professional boundaries can inadvertently disclose personal information that can impact on promotional prospects and so affect the career development of colleagues in the workplace (Maher, 1999).

The credibility of the facilitators and their skills in group facilitation are reiterated in the trauma therapy literature on CISD with the relationship ideally establishing between the debriefed and the debriefers: 'gentle, respectful interactions, clear verbal and non-verbal communication, clear co-leader leadership' (Pritchard, 2004: 57). The use of trained and registered clinicians is also highly recommended (Devilly and Cotton, 2003; Flannery and Everly, 2004; Suveg, 2007).

## Adaptation to context

Selecting participants for CISM interventions is considered to be of vital importance as only those who have been present at the critical incident should be involved in the debriefing (Lane, 1993; Maher, 1999; Pritchard, 2004). Therefore, a targeted approach to those who need the help most is reiterated from a trauma therapy perspective along with adaptation of CISD to suit differing work contexts (Morrison, 2007). For example, one US study discovered that there was 'limited applicability of the critical incident stress management model with a school age population' for trauma therapists in schools (Morrison, 2007: 771). A second shortcoming voiced by trauma therapists was that CISD needed to be adapted to the cultural background of the participants and for students, their developmental needs needed to be taken into account (Morrison, 2007). Attending to cultural, ethical and gender variables is important in the application and operation of CISM programmes (Morrison, 2007).

Adapting the language of CISD as an intervention to the audience's background, culture, gender and context is important to ensure that the organizational context surrounding the process is understood. Due to a gulf in understanding the culture of the audience, an external debriefer risks offending and alienating which may further traumatize those affected. In the case of working with children and young people in schools following a critical incident such as a sudden death of a classmate, for example, trauma therapists working in schools need to adapt the language of the debriefing models to evolve age-appropriate interventions (Morrison, 2007). Providing families with the tools and information for working with their own children affected by a critical incident may be more appropriate ethically than debriefing students in class with a facilitator. The former approach was one used during the 22 February 2011 earthquake in Christchurch, New Zealand, where teachers taught parents how to deal with traumatized students, in addition to various classroom interventions such as art therapy and creative writing to facilitate the expression of feelings among primary school students. An application of CISM models to work with families may, therefore, involve a systemic, strengths-based approach that capitalizes on naturally occurring support networks to use these resources as a first line of support and intervention following a critical incident rather than a formal debriefing by a trained facilitator.

## Strengths-based models of critical incident stress management

Strengths-based models and approaches are considered to be needed to supplement existing models of CISM (Pack, 2013, 2014b). Slawinski (2005) argues that promoting resilience needs to be the focus when considering psychological debriefing. She suggests combining strengths-based and ecological systems theories alongside CISM approaches and protocols to broaden the focus and the application of specific strategies such as psychological debriefing. Working with protective factors such as natural healing networks, cognitive coping strategies and self-esteem is suggested as these resources can be overlooked within CISM approaches. Furthermore, the combination of a strengths-based paradigm with ecological systems thinking may be more culturally sensitive as it can be adapted to the ways in which the individual already processes traumatic events within their social and community networks. Lim *et al.*, (2000) suggest that, when a critical event occurs, a 'circle of influence' exists for each person who is directly affected – starting with the helping professionals involved in the critical event, their family, friends, workplace, school, neighbourhood and community, state and nation. Therefore, any intervention following a critical event needs to occur on each of these levels within CISM programmes. Adamson (2006) concurs with these findings in her research as she proposes adequate preparation of students for the rigours of practice. She discovered in her doctoral research that job context, and in particular trauma therapists' interpersonal finesse in navigating complex and ambiguous situations in the workplace, is the major variable in determining interns' well-being in the workplace in the face of critical incidents. The rationale for this approach comes clearly from the evidence that

> a significant proportion of occupational stress comes not from specific events but from the environmental conditions that create ambiguities, tensions and conflict. Furthermore, these contextual pitfalls can undermine resilience in the event of critical incidents.
>
> (Adamson, 2006: 54–5)

The implications of this is that in trauma therapy, education preparation is needed to prepare new trauma therapy graduates to deal with the rigours of the practice environment (Adamson, 2006). This finding suggests the need for induction programmes for new trauma therapists to assist in their knowledge of different sections of the workplace. This knowledge can assist staff to access and use the range of services available.

## A targeted approach

Screening of individuals and their post-trauma histories is needed to refer those considered to more at risk of subsequent re-traumatization to appropriate debriefing and other services (Devilly and Cotton, 2004; Flannery and Everly, 2004; Suveg, 2007). For trauma therapists, the quality of their experiences in the organizational environment needs to be taken into consideration. For example, Regehr *et al.* (2004) conclude that trauma therapists employed in the field of child welfare need to be mindful of the effects of long-term workplace stressors in relation to predicting how they will likely respond to critical events. If critical events occur in an environment where there are chronic or long-term stressors that are ongoing, the intensity of the responses are likely to be increased (Regehr *et al.*, 2004). Workplace chronic stressors for trauma therapists include recording requirements, organizational change and working with difficult clients. Drawing on the cognitive self-development theory of McCann and Pearlman (1990), various protective factors enhancing resilience are identified (Regehr *et al.*, 2004). These protective factors include support by colleagues; individual cognitive constructs such as safety/trust and power and control; and 'incident factors' which refer to the length of time since the event and number of traumatic events encountered over the past year (Regehr *et al.*, 2004: 334).

Of these factors promoting individual trauma therapists' resilience, the organizational context is considered the most important factor (Regehr *et al.*, 2004). How well the organization operates in its day-to-day functioning suggests how effectively it will operate in a crisis mode as well as being indicative of the quality of care provided to clients and the level of care and support given to workers (Regel, 2007). This is a theme that I had discovered in researching vicarious traumatization and critical incidents among trauma therapists working as sexual abuse therapists (Pack, 2009) and that Maher (1999) identifies in the fire service. If the employing agency worked from an explicitly anti-oppressive position with management working collaboratively with workers, I discovered that this shared philosophy, together with clinical supervision and personal therapy enabled a smoother passage through critical events such as client suicide (Pack, 2009). The support of management in being involved in supporting employees to attend the critical incident management services was another variable in the programmes' success for the workers involved (Pack, 2014a).

## Conclusion

As there are many different interventions encompassed within CISM, there is the need for each of the many differing protocols to be more objectively evaluated by those not involved in the provision and facilitation of debriefings or coordinators of programmes (Lewis, 2003). It is recommended that the quality of the facilitation and the facilitators' own training and supervision be examined by independent researchers (Lewis, 2003). Further research is needed to determine which groups and for which kinds of critical incidents and in what context (individual or group) psychological debriefing is likely to be beneficial to participants

(Lewis, 2003). The role of context and in particular attention to the organizational setting is needed. Within and across organizations, contact with other CISM teams and programmes operating in the local area is recommended (Lane, 1993).

There is also an identified lack of research on the impact of debriefing on the debriefers themselves in terms of the resources they need to continue to sustain them in this role. The role of employer support to screen individuals vulnerable to post-trauma responses via employee assistance programmes and trained peer supporters is another area for further research.

## Attention to context, protective factors and strengths-based theories of resilience

The identification of protective factors such as social support and other personal resources needs to be considered alongside a theoretically grounded model of risk factors such as the moderating influences of age, gender, ethnicity and marital/socio-economic status (Donnelly and Siebert, 2009). Additionally, the influence of occupational risk factors needs to bring a contextual understanding to guide facilitators towards what is 'appropriate' intervention. What seems clear is that there is insufficient evidence that the CISM model and CISD protocol within that model is harmful and should be immediately suspended (Wagner, 2005). Overall, those workers who participate find that having an opportunity to discuss the emotional aftermath of events encountered in their work to be very supportive personally and professionally (Pack, 2009, 2014a, 2014b).

Perhaps the debates in the literature about the effectiveness of CISM ultimately will be informative of 'what works' when assisting professionals who deal with critical events (however these are defined), through a process of integrating experience. From my reviewing of the literature on models of CISM and CISD as an intervention, I note the existence of a conceptual 'holding space' out of which a more pragmatic definition of CISM models is forming. The new definition of 'what works' for trauma therapists in CISM involves a process of closer integration between the personal and professional values that the individual brings to practice. Central to this emerging new definition of CISM is the process of reflecting on the context (field of practice and employing organization) surrounding the triggering critical event and from that point of reference, evolving a new meaning about the event, one's identity as well as the context in which the incident has occurred. Inevitably this reflection involves the trauma therapist's whole self, based in personal and professional beliefs and values. The support of management involving proactive leadership of work teams needs to be part of an integrated CISM policy for trauma therapists out of which a range of interventions such as group and individual debriefing is offered on a voluntary or 'as needs' basis.

As Hibler (2000) asserts, the history of science replays constantly, making it difficult to determine the effect of what we consider to be 'innovations'. We need not be surprised then if the lessons learned will take time to integrate and the evolution of guidelines for the use of CISM developed.

## Checklist of components for a comprehensive CISM plan

1　Qualified and experienced facilitators of CISM programmes.
2　Full assessment of the individual's needs paying attention to protective factors such as social support and other personal resources/existing self-care.

3   Knowledge about Mitchell's multifaceted model comprising a staged approach.
4   Less formal peer support/supervision offered as an adjunct to formal CISM programmes.
5   Support of management involving proactive leadership of work teams.
6   A contextual understanding to guide facilitators towards what is 'appropriate' inter-
    vention. This shared philosophy, clinical supervision and personal therapy enabled a
    smoother passage through critical events such as client suicide.

(Pack, 2013, 2014a)

## Case study

Rose, one of the counsellor-participants, reflects on a critical incident involving her work
with a client that changed the way she worked subsequently with her clients. She also found
through working through this existential crisis, the experience of debriefing with her supervisor changed her life:

> Rose: The most stressful event was when the client completed counselling and then
> a couple of weeks later she committed suicide after travelling to live with a relation.
> Working through that and examining absolutely every aspect of my work and my being
> and then knowing that there wasn't anything that I could have changed. Although I did
> notice in my work from then on I was far more stringent in that question about people
> coming to me: whether they had desire to live or die and challenging, confronting that,
> which has really worked for me and for the clients.

> It put my life and therapy in perspective. I lost more of my idealism of thinking that I
> could change the world and at the same time I still really value therapy.

> [pause to enable reflection then the interview restarts at the participant's request]

> I'm just thinking of that occasion with just not having the answers, and that the wonder
> of the resilience of some people and being able to make sense and letting go of having
> to make sense of it. I think that is the big learning. Of accepting …

With time Rose decided she did not have 'all the answers' and in fact could hold and
tolerate the tragedy of what had occurred and how it affected her. She came to accept
her client's decision through a critical incident debriefing with her clinical supervisor.
While reflecting on the resilience of other clients who had decided to continue living and
with continued clinical supervision in an established and trustworthy relationship with her
supervisor, she was able to transcend her existential despair to continue practising as a
trauma therapist (Pack, 2014b).

Rose's story and this chapter might have evoked some of your own critical events, so the
following questions are offered to focus thinking on what more you wish to do to process
those events. For example, you might have reflected about an event in the past that has
triggered thinking about a similar case or theme in your caseload currently. This may be an
area to discuss in your clinical supervision or with a trusted colleague if there are recurring
themes and patterns linked to the critical incident(s) you have encountered on the job that are
still impacting your personal/professional life.

## Reflective questions on critical incidents encountered in practice and their impact

Thinking back over the length of your own career as a trauma therapist, what was the critical event that remains uppermost in your recollections?

- What happened?
- Who was involved?
- What were the central issues or dilemmas this event raised for you and others?
- Have there been any effects on you or your life/career subsequently?
- If there have been repercussions, what have these been and how do they affect you now?
- In retrospect, how would you have preferred to process the incident?
- What services singularly or in combination would have been helpful to you in dealing with the issues that arose for you (for example, defusing, debriefing, peer support or personal therapy, clinical supervision)?
- What help do you need to process critical incidents now and in the future?
- How might you obtain this help in the future within your organization or contracting arrangement?

## Websites offering information about CISM and CISD

Association of Traumatic Stress Specialists (ATSS)

A professional group of individuals from varying occupations committed to providing specialist trauma services, including CISM:

www.atss.info

Trauma information website with Mitchell *et al.*'s (2003) theorizing about CISD in the American context:

www.info-trauma.org/flash/media-e/mitchellCriticalIncidentStressDebriefing.pdf

This website aims to provide critical incident services to organizations and employees to assist in recovery from critical incidents. Provides a 24/7 chat line and freephone in Australia:

www.traumacentre.com.au/about-tca

International Critical Incident Stress Foundation (ICISF)

An international organization whose website offers training, contact and resources about CISM:

www.icisf.org

CISM peer support training in New Zealand:

www.cisresponse.com

# References

Adamson, C. (2006). Stress, trauma and critical incidents: The challenge for social work education. *ANZASW Social Work Review, 18* (4), 50–8.

Arendt, M. and Elklit, A. (2001). Effectiveness of psychological debriefing. *Acta Psychiatrica Scandinavica, 104* (6), 423–37.

Bell, J. L. (1995). Traumatic event debriefing: Service delivery designs and the role of social work therapy. *Social Work, 40* (1), 36–43.

Boudreaux, E. D. and McCabe, B. (2000). Emergency psychiatry: Critical incident stress management – I. Interventions and effectiveness. *Psychiatric Services, 51* (9), 1095–7.

Caine, R. M. and Ter-Bagdasarian, L. (2003). Advanced practice. Early identification and management of critical incident stress. *Critical Care Nurse, 23* (1), 59–65.

Deahl, M. (2000). Psychological debriefing: Controversy and challenge. *Australian and New Zealand Journal of Psychiatry, 34* (6), 929–39.

Deahl, M. P., Srinivasan, M., Jones, N., Neblett, C. and Jolly, A. (2001). Commentary: Evaluating psychological debriefing – Are we measuring the right outcomes? *Journal of Traumatic Stress, 14* (3), 527–9.

Devilly, G. J. and Cotton, P. (2003). Psychological debriefing and the workplace: Defining a concept, controversies and guidelines for intervention. *Australian Psychologist, 38* (2), 144–50.

Devilly, G. J. and Cotton, P. (2004). Caveat emptor, caveat venditor, and critical incident stress debriefing/management (CISD/M). *Australian Psychologist, 39* (1), 35–40.

Devilly, G. J., Gist, R. and Cotton, P. (2006). Ready! Fire! Aim! The status of psychological debriefing and therapeutic interventions: In the work place and after disasters. *Review of General Psychology, 10* (4), 318–45.

Donnelly, E. and Siebert, D. (2009). Occupational risk factors in the emergency medical services. *Prehospital and Disaster Medicine, 24* (5), 422–9.

Dyregrov, A. (1997). The process in psychological debriefings. *Journal of Traumatic Stress, 10* (4), 589–605.

Everly, G. S., Jr., Boyle, S. H. and Lating, J. M. (1999). The effectiveness of psychological debriefing with vicarious trauma: A meta-analysis. *Stress Medicine, 15* (4), 229–33.

Everly, G. S., Jr., Flannery, R. B., Jr., Eyler, V. and Mitchell, J. T. (2001). Sufficiency analysis of an integrated multicomponent approach to crisis intervention: Critical incident stress management. *Advances in Mind–Body Medicine, 17* (3), 174–81.

Figley, C. R. (Ed.). (1995). *Compassion fatigue: Coping with secondary traumatic stress disorder in those who treat the traumatized.* New York: Brunner/Mazel.

Flannery, R. B., Jr. and Everly, G. S., Jr. (2004). Critical incident stress management (CISM): Updated review of findings, 1998–2002. *Aggression and Violent Behavior, 9* (4), 319–29.

Freeman, D. G. H. and Carson, M. (2006). Developing workplace resilience: The role of the peer referral agent diffuser. *Journal of Workplace Behavioral Health, 22* (1), 113–21.

Galliano, S. (2002). Critical incident processing. *CPJ: Counselling and Psychotherapy Journal, 13* (6), 18–20.

Gist, R. and Devilly, G. J. (2002). Post-trauma debriefing: The road too frequently travelled. *Lancet, 360* (9335), 741–2.

Herman, J. (1992). *Trauma and recovery.* New York: Basic Books.

Hibler, R. J. (2000). In defense of defending what may not be so obvious in the CISD/CISM efficacy debates. *International Journal of Emergency Mental Health, 2* (4), 227.

Horn, J. M. (2002). Law enforcement and trauma. In Williams, M. B. and J. F. Sommer Jr., (Eds). *Simple and complex post-traumatic stress disorder: Strategies for comprehensive treatment in clinical practice* (pp. 311–23). New York: Hawthorne.

Irving, P. and Long, A. (2001). Critical incident stress debriefing following traumatic life experiences. *Journal of Psychiatric and Mental Health Nursing, 8* (4), 307–14.

Lane, P. S. (1993). Critical incident stress debriefing for health care workers. *Omega: Journal of Death and Dying, 28* (4), 301–15.

Lewis, S. J. (2003). Do one-shot preventive interventions for PTSD work? A systematic research synthesis of psychological debriefings. *Aggression and Violent Behavior*, *8* (3), 329–43.

Lim, J. J., Childs, J. and Gonsalves, K. (2000). Critical incident stress management. *AAOHN Journal*, *48* (10), 487–99.

McCann, I. L. and Pearlman, L. A. (1990). Vicarious traumatisation: A framework for understanding the psychological effects of working with victims. *Journal of Traumatic Stress*, *3* (1), 131–49.

MacNab, A., Sun, C. and Lowe, J. (2003). Randomized, controlled trial of three levels of critical incident stress intervention. *Prehospital and Disaster Medicine*, *18* (4), 367–71.

Maher, J. M. (1999). An exploration of the experience of critical incident stress debriefing on firefighters within a region of the New Zealand Fire Service (Unpublished master's thesis). Victoria University of Wellington, Wellington, New Zealand.

Mitchell, J. T. (1983). When disaster strikes: The critical incident stress debriefing process. *Journal of Emergency Medical Services*, *8* (1), 36–9.

Mitchell, J. T. (2004). A response to the Devilly and Cotton article, 'Psychological debriefing and the workplace …'. *Australian Psychologist*, *39* (1), 24–8.

Mitchell, A. M., Sakraida, T. J. and Kameg, K. (2003). Critical incident stress debriefing: Implications for best practice. *Disaster Management and Response*, *1* (2), 46–51.

Morrison, J. Q. (2007). Social validity of the critical incident stress management model for school-based crisis intervention. *Psychology in the Schools*, *44* (8), 765–77.

Pack, M. J. (2009). The body as a site of knowing: Sexual abuse therapists' experiences of stress and trauma. *Women's Study Journal*, *23* (2), 46–56. Retrieved from www.wsanz.org.nz (accessed 16 March 2016).

Pack, M. J. (2013). Critical incident stress management: A review of the literature with implications for social work. *International Social Work*, *56* (5), 608–27.

Pack, M. J. (2014a). The role of managers in critical incident stress management programmes: A qualitative study of New Zealand social workers. *Journal of Social Work Practice*, *28* (1), 43–57.

Pack, M. J. (2014b). Vicarious resilience: A multi-dimensional model of stress and trauma. *Affilia: Journal of Women and Social Work*, *29* (1): 18–29.

Plaggemars, D. (2000). EAPs and critical incident stress debriefing: A look ahead. *Employee Assistance Quarterly*, *16* (1–2), 77–95.

Pritchard, D. (2004). Critical incident stress and secondary trauma: An analysis of group process. *Groupwork: An Interdisciplinary Journal for Working with Groups*, *14* (3), 44–62.

Rabu, M., Moltu, C., Binder, P. and McLeod, J. (2015). How does practising psychotherapy affect the personal life of the therapist? A qualitative inquiry of senior therapists' experiences. *Psychotherapy Research*. doi: 10.1080/10503307.2015.1065354

Regehr, C., Hemsworth, D., Leslie, B., Howe, P. and Chau, S. (2004). Predictors of post traumatic distress in child welfare workers: A linear structural equation model. *Children and Youth Services Review*, *26* (4), 331–46.

Regel, S. (2007). Post-trauma support in the workplace: The current status and practice of critical incident stress management (CISM) and psychological debriefing (PD) within organizations in the UK. *Occupational Medicine*, *57* (6), 411–16.

Riddell, K. and Clouse, M. (2004). Comprehensive psychosocial emergency management promotes recovery. *International Journal of Emergency Mental Health*, *6* (3), 135–45.

Robertson, M., Humphreys, L. and Ray, R. (2004). Psychological treatments for posttraumatic stress disorder: Recommendations for the clinician based on a review of the literature. *Journal of Psychiatric Practice*, *10* (2), 106–18.

Robinson, R. (2000). Debriefing with emergency services: Critical incident stress management. In Raphael, B. and Wilson, J. (Eds). *Psychological debriefing: Theory, practice and evidence* (pp. 91–107). Cambridge: Cambridge University Press.

Robinson, R. (2004). Counterbalancing misrepresentations of critical incident stress debriefing and critical incident stress management. *Australian Psychologist*, *39* (1), 29–34.

Robinson, R. (2007). Commentary on 'Issues in the debriefing debate for the emergency services: Moving research outcomes forward'. *Clinical Psychology: Science and Practice*, *14* (2), 121–3.

Slawinski, T. (2005). A strengths-based approach to crisis response. *Journal of Workplace Behavioral Health, 21* (2), 79–88.

Spitzer, W. J. and Burke, L. (1993). A critical-incident stress debriefing program for hospital-based health care personnel. *Health and Social Work, 18* (2), 149–56.

Spitzer, W. J. and Neely, K. (1993). Critical incident stress: The role of hospital-based social work in developing a statewide intervention system for first-responders delivering emergency services. *Social Work in Health Care, 18* (1), 39–58.

Suveg, C. (2007). Implications of the debriefing debate for research and clinical practice. *Clinical Psychology: Science and Practice, 14* (2), 117–20.

Tuckey, M. R. (2007). Issues in the debriefing debate for the emergency services: Moving research outcomes forward. *Clinical Psychology – Science and Practice, 14* (2), 106–16.

van Emmerik, A. A. P., Kamphuis, J. H., Hulsbosch, A. M. and Emmelkamp, P. M. G. (2002). Single session debriefing after psychological trauma: A meta-analysis. *The Lancet, 360* (9335), 766–71.

Wagner, S. L. (2005). Emergency response service personnel and the critical incident stress debriefing debate. *International Journal of Emergency Mental Health, 7* (1), 33–41.

# Chapter 8 The search for self and the search beyond self

## The role of connection to spirituality, nature and community in self-care

I think that because there are so many personal demands on you in doing this work, I can't imagine what it would be like to not be plugged into something greater than me. Part of my degree was in religious studies so I'm interested in the essence of all the traditions. I'm not a practising Christian at all. I'm not a practising Buddhist but there are elements of all the religions I practise.

*Sophia talking about what spirituality means to her in the context of her practice as a trauma therapist*

### Introduction

In this chapter, the related themes of spirituality, nature and connection to community are explored as protective factors that build resilience among trauma therapists (Pack, 2014). Reference to body and the mind–body connection was part of the journey of discovery the counsellor-participants embarked upon in caring for themselves and others (Pack, 2009). This chapter suggests both that vicarious traumatization acts as a rite of passage and that its understanding is essential to the development of personal resources required to practise in the field as a trauma therapist. These cycles of personal reflection and development of the relationship between self and other, client and self, and spirituality I have referred to as 'the search for self', and 'the search beyond self'. These are connected processes in which the trauma therapist is engaged. These processes, over time, enable therapists to make sense of their work, themselves and the societal forces that colour the environment in which trauma and therapy take place (Pack, 2004, 2009). New sources of knowledge are developed out of this search which can be used as a resource from which trauma therapists practise and nurture themselves and others both personally and professionally (Pack, 2014).

The current chapter, building on earlier theory development (Pack, 2004, 2009), suggests that resilience like vicarious traumatization stems from trauma therapists' empathetic engagement in the traumatic disclosures from their clients. Engagement in traumatic client disclosures and therapists' responses to them is, paradoxically, both the source of vicarious traumatization and the means of building resilience (Pack, 2014). As outlined in Chapter 2, in my own research with sexual abuse therapists, this existential despair was a key feature of the first five years of practice that needed to be actively planned for (Pack, 2010). Empathetic engagement with the client's traumatic material led to an overriding sense of dissonance or disjuncture which jettisoned therapists into an unknown zone which I have conceptualized as prompting a search for meaning in a liminal space or a space of not knowing but becoming (Pack, 2014). Aspects of this disjunction were manifested in physical sensations (heart palpations or feeling as though one was having a heart attack, a variety of breathing problems and dizziness).

These kinds of experiences, while also likely evidence of traumatic transference (Herman, 1992), prompted a deeper existential search involving two related components – the 'search for self' involving the reformulation of personal and professional identities and the 'search beyond self' which is a deeper search for a reformulated spirituality or connection to higher sources of knowing through personal growth (Pack, 2014).

For the counsellor-participants interviewed, the search for inner strength through spirituality was connected with a growing disillusionment with hierarchy and patriarchal structures (Pack, 2004, 2014). An awareness of abuse in the church brought about a search for alternative sources of the intangible aspects of life. 'Spirituality' was increasingly referred to as belonging to a group working towards the collective good of humanity. The counsellor-participants developed an awareness of being connected to a greater source of being, which replaced or modified earlier-held beliefs. These evolving beliefs established a new way of being and relating to the world and others. These revised beliefs established a context for continuing to practise as a trauma therapist. Rose explains how she has integrated her developing sense of spirituality with her involvement in the church in which she was raised:

> Rose: My spirituality has grown and changed … a lot of the dogma doesn't fit with my beliefs any more … I value, currently and for the last 20 years, being part of a community of people with similar spiritual beliefs. I'm currently part of two communities, one a community of women whom I've been involved with; two, a group of eight for about 20 years and that's a group which is based around the Catholic spirituality. Their work is to carry out spiritual retreat work.
>
> (Pack, 2014)

## Spirituality: the lived experience of being a trauma therapist

The spirituality discussed by the counsellor-participants drew from theories of feminist embodiment (such as those theories developed by Irigaray, 1980, 1993) and trauma-informed practice and recovery (Herman, 1992, 2010).

Reference to the theories of feminist writers such as Herman (1992, 2010), who views trauma therapy as a political act of witnessing, goes beyond what is conventionally thought of as psychodynamic psychotherapy. Herman (1992, 2010) has identified three stages in the recovery process from trauma: the establishment of safety of the survivor; remembrance and mourning; and the reconstruction of personal narratives. Once safety is secured, feminist empowerment principles guide each stage of the recovery process. Retelling the narrative of the traumatic event assists the traumatic memories to be assimilated into the survivor's life story. Empowerment continues to guide this stage of recovery with the survivor controlling the pace and details shared with the therapist. The final stage of therapy involves the survivor rebuilding the assumptions and beliefs that have been damaged by trauma through reconnection involving developing a new sense of self; relationship and meaning in life in the present; and looking forward to the future (Herman, 1992, 2010).

To begin to explain the meaning-making that occurs for trauma counsellors, a parallel process of healing is embarked upon. To understand this parallel process of recovery, I also drew on theories of embodied experience from the French essentialist feminists, exemplified in the writings of Irigaray (1980, 1993). Theorists writing from an essentialist feminist position such as Irigaray value the idea of women's autonomy and difference based on the lived experience of the female body. Irigaray critiques ideas that are prefaced on 'gender' as bodily sameness and views the goal of women's attainment of equality within male-stream systems as failing to liberate women from the patriarchal discourses (Pack, 2014).

Language is a major concern of Irigaray and the French essentialist feminists. To use language indiscriminately is unintentionally to confirm and promote patriarchal thinking (Irigaray, 1980, 1993). Irigaray considers that we need to find new ways of writing about women's experience in an attempt to free language from patriarchal thought in which it has become enmeshed. She develops discourses that suggest that women's ways of knowing, based on the lived experience of the female body, are important sources of wisdom. For example, Irigaray interviews Dr Helen Rouch, a scientist who has reformulated our understanding of the relationship between mother and child in utero. Dr Rouch describes the placenta as existing in a symbiotic rather than the parasitic relationship described in medical discourses (Irigaray, 1993). Irigaray, drawing from such reformulations, challenges the duality and sense of separation based in the predominant scientific discourses. In so doing, Irigaray brings direct, bodily experience within the realms of what counts as 'knowledge'.

Being aware of one's own identity is a starting point within which trauma therapists can centre their practice. The importance of reclaiming one's own narrative when it has been marginalized, limited or lost for whatever reason, is akin to the re-writing of history from the perspective of first nations peoples who have experienced the effects of Western colonization. From this perspective, identity is both a guide to action and a process for deconstructing the dominant discourses. Chapter 4 of this book illustrated this theme with examples of re-authoring from the counsellor-participants and from my own practice.

For example, Linda, a counsellor-participant, looked at the process of colonization of New Zealand by Pākehā as being a parallel process to the abuse and violence experienced by women. Linda developed her thinking about the connections between abuse and colonization as a result of her involvement in feminism and, more recently, in coming to identify what being Māori meant for her personally. She drew on this knowledge to guide her practice with clients who identified as Māori. In the following excerpt from her interview, she talks of her knowledge of her own identity and *whākāpapa* [genealogy] within Māoridom, specifically that identifying her *iwi* [tribe], *hāpu* [sub-tribe] and *whānau* [extended family] became a knowledge base used in her work as a therapist. She discovered that she changed her approach to therapy as she began incorporating her newfound identity as a Māori woman in her work as a therapist with trauma survivors:

> Linda: Originally I think I was coming very much from a feminist perspective. The cultural aspect for me has come alongside my own personal development in terms of being Māori because when I first got involved in this work, I was struggling in terms of my own identity. So it was a parallel process, really. So for me, as I have become more whole, in terms of being a Māori woman, I've developed a bigger-picture understanding of how this area of work relates to Māori in particular because I very rarely work with non-Māori. The identity issue is really important. So if we look at that it would be about people making contact with their *whānau* and exploring their *whākāpapa* and finding out where they come from and their particular *iwi* and to be able to go home, being able to know where their *marae* [tribal community/meeting place] is.

Holistic and more relational therapies enabled the counsellor-participants to position themselves in alternative theoretical frameworks. Moments of crisis in therapy were often first noticed by the counsellors as a series of bodily sensations. These signs became constitutive of meaning in working with clients who had been sexually abused. It was also informative of the process and transference within therapy (Pack, 2009).

To understand the language of their clients and of their own suffering, the counsellors' awareness of various bodily sensations became a guide to connecting with the unspoken content of trauma that the client communicated through affect and often through impulsive actions, including situations involving self-harm. To understand the content of this non-verbal material, the counsellors found that they needed to connect with the experience of their own bodies. As a means of making this connection, a variety of bodywork theories such as Vipassanā meditation and Hakomi were used. Bodywork theories such as Hakomi, a branch of psychotherapy informed by Eastern philosophies, aim to bring the mind and the body into a greater alignment. These therapies direct attention to bodily awareness and use techniques such as meditation and mindfulness activities around the experience of the body and connect these experiences to what is occurring in the mind. By reformulating their own mind–body awareness as a source of knowledge, the counsellor-participants discovered that they were able, over time, to transcend the dissociation that accompanied work with sexual abuse survivors to more effectively engage with clients while avoiding the worst effects of vicarious traumatization.

## Mindfulness practices

Along with identity and genealogy, and the notion of re-authoring, activities such as mindfulness and being in nature have been found conducive to managing vicarious traumatization (Martinek, 2010). Mindfulness is a Buddhist practice whose origins can be traced to the Four Noble Truths. To remain grounded while immersed in traumatic disclosure from clients, mindfulness, as defined in awareness of self and understanding of self, is necessary to maintain equilibrium as a therapist (Pearlman and Saakvitne, 1995). More recently, studies of being in wilderness have found this to have positive impact on those who are working as therapists with trauma (Martinek, 2010). A recent study's findings support the notion that being in nature brings opportunities for harmony and healing with oneself as opportunities for felt connections between self and the natural world are made possible (Martinek, 2010). Many of the counsellor-participants went on retreats in rural locations, many relocating permanently to live in a closer relationship with natural surroundings in small town communities (Pack, 2010). This was a lifestyle choice made clearer by an appreciation of belonging in a local/rural community, with an underlying green philosophy. This connection with the earth was described by a partner of one of the counsellor-participants in the following way: 'I'm thinking in terms of the lifestyle we've often talked about that we could have on a farm. Jill would like to be more connected to the land and literally to be there for it …'.

Beth, another of the counsellor-participants, discussed being near the sea as restorative to her spirituality as there she had a nurturing sense of the presence of important figures in her life who are now deceased. Giving thanks and gratitude to all beings was part of her daily routine:

> Beth: The spiritual practices that are important that have sustained me over the last year or so are getting in touch with nature. Things like walking on the beach, like enjoying the fabulous garden I've been living in and beginning each day with a personal meditational prayer-like ritual. And being thankful for life – that's something that is very important to me that I have practised a lot which maintains myself for work and for life generally. And it includes remembering the people who've been in my life who have died and who are still with me …

But how and why is a focus on connection to spirituality, nature and community important as an aspect of self-care for trauma therapists? Again it is necessary to return to four of the core concepts introduced in Chapter 1: 'vicarious traumatisation' (McCann and Pearlman, 1990; Pearlman and Saakvitne, 1995); 'secondary traumatic stress' (Figley, 1995; Stamm, 1996); 'traumatic transference' (Herman, 1992); and 'compassion fatigue' (Figley, 1995).

## Returning to the vicarious traumatization literature

To recap on the concepts and how they can be distinguished, which were outlined in Chapter 2, vicarious traumatization refers to how therapists' cognitive changes and values encapsulated in constructivist self-development theory are transformed with continued exposure to traumatic material over time (McCann and Pearlman, 1990).

Secondary traumatic stress as defined by Figley (1995) and Stamm (1996) refers to the phenomenon of post-traumatic stress impacting professional workers who deal with trauma in a parallel way to the clients they are assisting who are experiencing PTSD. This parallel process between client and worker can precipitate a secondary kind of post-traumatic stress for the professionals who deal with trauma, for example, when paramedics assist clients in emergency situations. When secondary traumatic stress is in evidence, practitioners can experience the phenomenon of 'compassion fatigue' which is akin to a triggering of compassion leading to a form of professional burnout (Figley, 1996). This phenomenon may arise suddenly (which is unlike vicarious traumatization which is thought to be cumulative and increase with exposure over time) and be typified by emotional exhaustion, hypervigilance, avoidance and withdrawal. Unlike vicarious traumatization, compassion fatigue does not specifically include changes to beliefs, cognitions and world view. Secondary traumatic stress is conceptualized as the process through which 'compassion fatigue' occurs (Figley, 1996).

Psychotherapists dealing with traumatized clients, due to the long-term nature of the work with complex presentations, are usually witness to trauma that is transformative of core belief structures and world view (Pearlman and Saakvitne, 1995). A distinguishable kind of countertransference that relates specifically to working with trauma has been termed 'traumatic transference' (Herman, 1992). While Freud is acknowledged as the originator of the term 'transference', Herman (1992) applied the impact of trauma in relation to the unique responses triggered in the therapist's past from engagement with trauma from clients in the present. When traumatic transference is experienced, past psychological wounds once healed are again thought to be rekindled by this engagement.

Taken together these terms (vicarious traumatization, secondary traumatic stress and compassion fatigue) are referred to as 'the cost of caring' (Figley, 1996), sharing some common features but also some differences. A meta-analysis of studies dealing with vicarious traumatization and secondary traumatic stress was undertaken in 2006 to see if there is convincing evidence that the impact of the work in the trauma field has identifiable risks and hazards for practitioners (Baird and Kracen, 2006). The problem the authors identified was that the field of vicarious traumatization and secondary traumatic stress was only ten years old at that time with many of the empirical research studies being exploratory (Baird and Kracen, 2006). However, despite limitations with the methodology of the reviewed studies, the authors found that there was 'persuasive evidence' that the amount of exposure to traumatic material was correlated in the development of secondary traumatic stress. Having a personal history of trauma was found significant in the development of vicarious traumatization which concurs with the earlier studies reviewed (Baird and Kracen, 2006: 184).

More recent developments have been the term 'soul pain' to describe a spiritual pain that is thought to stem from seeing cruelty inflicted by one human being on another without the witness being able to intervene to stop it (Jirek, 2015: 2). Based on in-depth interviews, 29 domestic violence shelter workers discussed numerous physical symptoms after completing a day's work, including recurrent and disturbing dreams involving themes of abuse in situations of no-escape (Jirek, 2015). As well as emotional numbing and detachment, staff members reported sadness which upon further probing revealed a sense of 'spiritual unrest' linked to anger, powerlessness to make change, and existential despair and hopelessness. In such a climate, the workers reported a tendency to 'lose faith in the world' (Jirek 2015: 15–16). Such crises lead to a search for meaning that involves the search for self and identity, and a related search involving the intangible aspects of life known as 'spirituality'.

## The search for self

In this section of the results, the counsellor-participants described a search for self that was generated by their engagement in the traumatic narratives of their clients. These experiences were sometimes described as 'directly traumatizing' or 'vicariously traumatizing' or a combination of both. What was 'traumatizing' was conceptualized as a sense of 'disjuncture' with oneself and others. The effects of trauma on self and other relationships described in the vicarious traumatization theory align with this finding (Pearlman and Saakvitne, 1995). Bodily and emotional manifestations of this 'disjuncture' were described by the counsellor-participants which fit with essentialist feminist theories of embodiment (Irigaray, 1980, 1993), awareness of which became a source of alternative ways of making meaning from experience. Sophia, one of the counsellor-participants, thought there was an earthquake in her counselling rooms when she was seeing a client when the trauma was unspoken:

> Sophia: I would sometimes feel the floor shaking under me. I actually went as far as having my heart checked and it was fine. I began to notice that when there was a really strong emotional content that wasn't being expressed like if someone was saying something that was really big, I would feel it in my body and it would make me feel dizzy or faint or my heart speed up or whatever. I learned how to work with that as soon as I figured out what was going on. Then I'd know what kind of questions to ask to elicit whatever was coming up. But it definitely has a physical effect on my body.

## Reformulating personal and professional identities

Re-authoring personal narratives as the counsellor-participants worked with abuse survivors was part of the search for self (Pack, 2014). The counsellor-participants had an appreciation of how their proximity to survivors of trauma and sexual assault imbued their own personal and professional narratives. One of the counsellor-participants, Sally, discussed the difficulty of communicating the hope that inspired their continued involvement in sexual abuse therapy to others. Framing her roles in life in new ways was important to her in relationship with friends who were not a part of the counselling profession:

> Sally: I don't actually often tell people what I do. I'll tell them about my teaching work but if it's new people and they say: 'what do you do?' I'll usually say: 'I tutor and do counselling and grow flowers'. And because it's all together they can pick out which one they want and they don't usually pick out counselling of course [laugh]. It gives a balance.

In order to reconstruct their identities, the counsellor-participants ventured out of the known into uncharted territory. Their experiences mirrored the dilemma feminists highlight of the need for women to move into areas of traditional male power with the intention of transforming them and the need for women to redefine these same areas with their own experience of their suffering and powerlessness (Irigaray, 1980, 1993). What was considered as 'traumatizing' was the assessment role that was required, which was seen as conflicting with best efforts in therapy. Audrey, another of the counsellor-participants, decided to leave the statutory department to establish her own private practice, but kept being offered incentives to stay. She decided to combine roles as a stepping stone to leaving to establish her own private practice:

> Audrey: It was having to stop having the focus on assessment and broaden my skills because I thought if I stay in this too long, if I stay in this for four to five years, I thought, that is not very good for my career, so I will broaden it. Which happened for the first couple of months and then I did one assessment and they saw that I could do it and they needed more, so I just got hundreds of assessments. I still kept my private therapy practice going though.
>
> (Pack, 2014)

The search for inner strength through the growth of spirituality was connected with the counsellor-participants' increasing disillusionment with hierarchy and patriarchal structures. They developed an awareness of being connected to a greater source of being which replaced earlier-held religious beliefs. These revised beliefs established a context for continuing to practise as a sexual abuse counsellor. A consultant to the present study, who wished to be known as George, was a minister of religion prior to his decision to train to become a psychotherapist. In a similar way, four of the other counsellor-participants had left their respective churches as ministers of religion and moved into counselling. George saw this movement into therapy and away from the church as 'a natural progression':

> George: People ask me why I left and I say it was interfering with my spiritual growth. The straw that finally broke the camel's back for me was sitting in church with a wife and three daughters and finding them invisible. They just didn't fit in the system. There was no language for them. It was a total male structure … So it was a real disappointment about having a structure that I thought was damaging to women. It was a huge motivating factor to leaving the church with having a wife and three daughters who are all feminists.
>
> (Pack, 2010)

## The search beyond self: spirituality and personal growth

In this section of the findings, the theme of spirituality and connection to community is explored as building resilience among the counsellor-participants interviewed.

The search for inner strength through spirituality seemed to be connected with a growing disillusionment with hierarchy and patriarchal structures as illustrated above by the excerpt from my interview with George. An awareness of abuse in the church brought about a search for alternative sources of the intangible aspects of life. 'Spirituality' was increasingly referred to as belonging to a group working towards the collective good of humanity. The counsellor-participants developed an awareness of being connected to a greater source of being, which replaced or modified earlier-held beliefs. These evolving beliefs established a new way of being and relating to the world and others.

For those therapists who had an awareness of sexual misconduct, male oppression and abuse within the conventional church systems they had worked and worshipped within, there was a desire to leave the existing hierarchies to begin a new life. For one of the counsellor-participants, being involved in abuse counselling within the church where she was a minister was 'the last straw':

> Sally: I'm not going to be a part of the church again because in a way it is like being stuck in there for so long, it's sort of like being in this domestic violence sort of thing: I keep coming back for more. I won't be a part of it. I was also part of the sexual misconduct advisory group within the church and I stuck with that because I thought I could make a difference. But in fact I've just resigned from that. That is partly why I am not in the church any more. I think it is abusive to think of women as being lesser in some way. To me, that is abusive as well as actual physical/sexual abuse.

For the women who decided to leave the church of which they were either members or ministers, the increasing number of sexual abuse cases coming to light within the church formed the background to their decision to move away. Frustration at trying to change the system from within to make it more accessible and supportive towards women became an aim the participants did not think was realistic. Sally, herself a minister, explains:

> Sally: I guess in the end I got very disillusioned with the church. And so a part of that, not the whole, just a small part, I was involved in the area where people were coming out about sexual abuse cases within the church. And that was the last straw I think [pause to consider]. Yes it was. And it was a period of change for me but it seemed like I was already moving away from the church and then just to become aware of the abuse, of actual cases that were going on. One was aware that there had been abuse in a wide sense, but to actually now hear specific cases. I thought: I don't actually want to be part of this abusive situation … they were all little points to saying: you've got choice, you've tried to change the system or you can actually leave the system. And I decided: no, I would rather leave. I think I have spent too long trying to change systems, so let's have a break.

Through engagement with traumatic disclosures, the counsellor-participants returned to their own corporeality. The experience of vicarious trauma had disconnected them from their sources of sustenance in a parallel way to their clients. Both counsellors and their clients are brought into a greater awareness of their corporeality as they are living within male-stream discourses through these experiences. Irigaray (1980, 1993) and other feminists writing from an essentialist feminist perspective have suggested that the place of the unspeakable (the body) is also a place of desire, celebration and joy. There are also emancipatory stories of the body that are resistant or even impervious to trauma. These are narratives of the body that are resilient to living within the predominant discourses while, simultaneously, learning to live outside them. The transformation of the body as 'voiceless' to the remaking of the body through reformulated discourses creates a counter-culture within the predominant patriarchal discourses and returns subjectivity or voice to the speaker (Pack, 2009, 2014).

The development of a spirituality that returned counsellor-participants to their subjectivity also allowed the counsellors interviewed to help their clients to reclaim their voice and so re-author their identity. Sometimes personal experience of abuse jettisoned the counsellor-participants into their own therapy which brought meaning to their personal experiences. The political act of witnessing (Herman, 1992) became an important means of caring for oneself as the work nurtured a growing sense of one's own survivorship and personal growth. Ellen, one of the consultant therapists interviewed, explained. Her growing sense of spirituality arising from her work with dissociative clients had grown now that she saw her resources being more 'internal':

> Ellen: I realize, too, that my work with sexual abuse has been balanced by clients who are on their own journey of self-discovery. In that time I realize, too, where I might have a focus of authority which is external, when I first began working in this area. I have shifted now to much more having an internal focus of authority. I can still be extroverted when required but I would say that my resources are now internal. So that has come from working with clients who have to find their own internal resources. They have been abused, but they need to find their own source of life within. I guess that has been their gift to me.

Balancing work in the therapy field with social change and action has been recommended as an antidote to vicarious traumatization (Pearlman and Saakvitne, 1995). The counsellor-participants concurred with this recommendation.

For a participant who wished to be known as Hayley, counselling survivors was seen as a natural outworking of her values and personal philosophy that had been shaped by her own abuse experiences:

> Hayley: In terms of trauma work, the personal experience was one of the pieces and positive experiences I had in terms of receiving counselling. If I go back even further to think of why I was so much into the rights issue then it would be as well living in different cultures and seeing at a young age people who had a lot more rights than other people. So that has always been there for me in terms of rights and justice issues.

What these counsellor stories of practice suggest is the importance of remaining relational with clients until they have integrated the awareness gained in therapy. However, in the cases discussed as 'difficult', there were impediments to achieving this goal that included continuing client self-harm, victimization and suicide. Referring to feminist theories of the body to understand the counsellor-participants' narratives suggests another way of working with clients and with the reformulation of material that is 'hard' for counsellors to hear. The challenge faced by the counsellors is one of reconnecting with their own subjectivity to enable clients to reconnect with theirs. To do this, the counsellor-participants actively pursued sources of knowledge that allowed them to re-invent themselves using the lived experience of the body (Pack, 2009, 2014).

## Conclusion

This chapter suggests that vicarious traumatization both acts as a rite of passage and is essential to the development of the coping resources and self-efficacy required to practise in the field as a sexual abuse therapist. These cycles of personal reflection and the development of the relationship between self and other, client and self, and spirituality I have referred to as 'the search for self', and 'the search beyond self' (Pack, 2014). These are connected processes in which the trauma therapist is engaged. These processes, over time, enable therapists to make sense of their work, themselves and the societal forces that colour the environment in which sexual abuse and therapy take place (Pack, 2004, 2009). This new source of knowledge is then developed out of this search and can be used as a resource from which sexual abuse therapists practise and nurture themselves and others both personally and professionally.

## Case study: Rose's reformulated insights about her spirituality

In closing, I will leave the final words to Rose, one of the counsellor-participants. In this excerpt from an interview, Rose summarizes how the movement away from organized religion into spirituality of her own making assists her in work as a therapist working in the field of abuse and trauma:

> Rose: Yes, I think the work at first felt all-encompassing. And now the work feels balanced in my life far more. I think over the years as a therapist it feels like cutting through the crap of institutions and dogma and feeling the frustration that it takes many years for institutions to come on board with new ideas, with theory and social change. And in a way I struggle to stay with part of an institution and then made the decision that I could live more freely and be more alive free of institutional life …
>
> I've experienced with my knowledge of what the impact of abuse has been and the effect of power and control; then being close to an institution that doesn't necessarily examine itself fast enough, where it tends to be the male-dominated systems, the change is just not fast enough. It's been easier to get on with my own life, my own being away from those institutions. I have now given up on trying to bring about change within the institution. At the same time I'm hugely supportive of those who continue to stay within and work for change.

---

### Questions for reflection

- What are the sources of spirituality that are important in your own life?
- Are there any areas you wish to develop? List three next steps you wish to make in this area of your life.
- When you experience the dissonance between personal values and professional experiences, what core beliefs and values are you aware of? Create a list.
- How might you mediate or address the gap between the two? Again jot down your ideas and next steps.

---

## Useful resources for mindfulness training: teachers, retreat centres and books

Spiritual writers such as Ajahn Chah (*Mindful Way*, nd) discuss being in nature as a way of developing harmony with onself and what is in the present (Ajahn Chah, nd). To come to this awareness, meditation in various forms is recommended as the means to living a conscious life. Meditation courses are easily accessible providing the tools for cultivating awareness and the Buddhist virtues of compassion, sympathetic joy for the success of others and *mettā* or universal lovingkindness. Here are some online resources for readers wishing to learn more about meditation as a means of exploring the deeper realities of being:

Ajahn Chah *Mindful Way*: www.youtube.com/watch?v=qu7mtlbVBOA

Excerpts from the BBC documentary *The Mindful Way* which show Luang Por Chah (also available in full on video.google.com), briefly featuring the young Ajahn Liam who was later nominated by Luang Por Chah to lead Wat Pah Pong and continues to do so.

For more video, audio and text see:

www.watnongpahpong.org
www.ajahnchah.org

## Insight Meditation Society

An international network of meditation retreat centres offering refuge and guidance in meditation known as Vipassanā (mindfulness practice) and *mettā* (lovingkindness meditation):

www.dharma.org
www.insightmeditationaustralia.org
www.jackkornfield.com

A practitioner for over 40 years, Jack Kornfield is one of the key teachers to introduce mindfulness and Vipassanā meditation to the West. His approach emphasizes compassion, lovingkindness and the profound path of mindful presence, all offered in simple, accessible ways in his books, CDs, classes and retreats.

## Mindfulness apps

HeadSpace:

www.headspace.com/headspace-meditation-app

Stop, breathe and think:

http://stopbreathethink.org

You can type in how you are feeling and the app will give you a few options for practices and you can track how you are going and which practices worked for you.

The *Saturday Evening Post* Top 10 Apps for Meditation:

www.saturdayeveningpost.com/2013/08/14/health-and-family/tech/meditation-apps.html

Simply Being:

https://itunes.apple.com/us/app/simply-being-guided-meditation/id347418999?mt=8

Smiling mind (created in Melbourne by Monash Mindfulness):

http://smilingmind.com.au

Take a break, free guided meditation for stress relief:

https://itunes.apple.com/au/app/take-break!-guided-meditations/id453857236?mt=8

Free guided meditation, 'Take a Break' for Android:

https://play.google.com/store/apps/details?id=com.meditationoasis.takeabreak&hl=en

133

## Free guided meditations

UCLA:

http://marc.ucla.edu/body.cfm?id=22

Guided meditation on Youtube:

www.youtube.com/watch?v=aS5QpPRFdbg

Guided meditation with Thich Nhat Hanh:

www.youtube.com/watch?v=ehhzQq7cIuc

How to meditate:

http://tarabrach.com/howtomeditate.html

Sounds True – weekly wisdom:

Free teachings on meditation and other areas of wellness:

www.soundstrue.com/store/weeklywisdom

## Activities and self-care exercises

Meditation Lab, University of New South Wales

https://student.unsw.edu.au/meditation-lab

On this website there are some exercises documenting some of the classes in the Meditation Lab in a podcast from the director:

www.community.nsw.gov.au/docswr/_assets/main/lib100056/fact_sheet_11_self_care_&_mindfulness.pdf

http://kspope.com/ethics/self-care.php

http://socialwork.buffalo.edu/resources/self-care-starter-kit/self-care-assessments-exercises/exercises-and-activities.html#title_5

## Meditation/mindfulness teachers

Jon Kabat-Zinn is credited with developing mindfulness-based stress reduction (MBSR):

Mindfulness with Jon Kabat-Zinn:

www.youtube.com/watch?v=3nwwKbM_vJc

Mindfulness meditation taster (12 minutes) with Jon Kabat-Zinn:

www.youtube.com/watch?v=D5Fa50oj45s

Thich Nhat Hanh is a Vietnamese monk who has written widely on mindfulness and Buddhism:

*The miracle of mindfulness: The classic guide to meditation by the world's most revered master.* London: Rider, 2008.

Thich Nhat Hanh: 'Mindfulness as a foundation for health: Talks at Google':

www.youtube.com/watch?v=Ijnt-eXukwk

Pema Chodron is a Western Tibetan Buddhist nun:
*The wisdom of no escape: How to love yourself and your world.* London: Element, 2003.

## *Self-care/spirituality/mindfulness resources recommended by the counsellor-participants*

Books and resources that may be useful/helpful … The work of Peter A. Levine, *Waking the Tiger: Healing Trauma*; *In an Unspoken Voice*; *How the Body Releases Trauma and Restores Goodness*; *Trauma through a Child's Eyes*; *Awakening the Ordinary Miracle of Healing*.

The work of Dr Bessel van der Kolk, including trauma-centred yoga and healing, here is a link to the clinic in Brookline, MA: www.traumacenter.org/research/research_landing.php

I'd also highly recommend *Sitting Together* by Ron Siegel, Susan Pollak and Tom Pedulla, which is a book for clinicians, but has many wonderful practices and a lot on working with trauma.

I've heard good things about this resource and book: http://traumastewardship.com. It's received good reviews from Thich Nhat Hanh and Jack Kornfield, and people I know who have used it have also found it useful.

All mindfulness practices are helpful for professional self-care as they all lower stress levels – it's like asking what type of physical exercise might be helpful – in general, whatever exercise the person is most likely to actually do. Having said that, those mindfulness exercises that strengthen 'this is me, that is them' can be especially helpful for potential compassion fatigue situations. These might fall into a couple of different categories depending on how one is taking on the stress of the other. Lovingkindness meditation, equanimity meditation, mindful movement or any exercise (to release stress from our own body), self-compassion practices (to understand and be with our own suffering) and especially staying close to one's own emotional life through mindfulness of emotions/feelings can all be particularly helpful.

If I had to pick one practice it would be mindfulness of current physical/mental/emotional experience to stay close to one's self in a kind and friendly way and not get dissociated from oneself; and then a second practice that is the most centring/grounding for each person (will be different for each person), making sure there is a healthy dose of self-compassion in the mix. If someone is not doing physical exercise, then mindful movement is essential. It is next to impossible to avoid eventual burnout and compassion fatigue if one is not regularly releasing stress from the body.

Any of the exercises from the Mindful Self-Compassion course would be helpful. See centerformsc.org or *The Mindful Way through Self-Compassion* by Chris Germer. Here is a study that reviewed mindfulness apps. It doesn't evaluate effectiveness just reviews content: http://mhealth.jmir.org/2015/3/e82/?trendmd-shared=0

# References

Baird, K. and Kracen, A. (2006). Vicarious traumatization and secondary traumatic stress: A research synthesis, *Counselling Psychology Quarterly*, *19* (2), 181–8. doi: 10.1080/09515070600811899

Figley, C. R. (1995). *Compassion fatigue*, New York: Brunner/Mazel.

Herman, J. (1992). *Trauma and recovery*. New York: Basic Books.

Herman, J. (2010). *Trauma and recovery: From domestic abuse to political terror*. London: Pandora.

Irigaray, L. (1980). When our lips speak together (C. Burke, Trans.). *Signs: Journal of Women in Culture and Society*, *6* (1), 69–79.

Irigaray, L. (1993). *Je, tu, nous: Toward a culture of difference* (A. Martin, Trans.). London: Routledge.

Jirek, S. L. (2015). Soul pain: The hidden toll of working with survivors of physical and sexual violence. *Sage Open*, *5* (13), 1–13.

McCann, I. L. and Pearlman, L. A. (1990). Vicarious traumatisation: A framework for understanding the psychological effects of working with victims. *Journal of Traumatic Stress*, *3* (1), 131–49.

Martinek, J. (2010). Embracing wilderness to heal counsellor vicarious trauma (Unpublished master's thesis). Alberta: University of British Columbia.

Pack, M. J. (2004). Sexual abuse counsellors' responses to stress and trauma: A social work perspective. *New Zealand Journal of Counselling, 25* (2), 1–17.

Pack, M. J. (2009). The body as a site of knowing: Sexual abuse therapists' experiences of stress and trauma. *Women's Study Journal, 23* (2), 46–56.

Pack, M. (2010). Career themes in the lives of sexual abuse counsellors. *New Zealand Journal of Counselling, 30* (2), 75–92.

Pack, M. (2014). Vicarious resilience: A multilayered model of stress and trauma. *Affilia: Journal of Women and Social Work, 29* (1), 18–29.

Pearlman, L. A. and Saakvitne, K. W. (1995). *Trauma and the therapist: Countertransference and vicarious traumatisation in psychotherapy with incest survivors*. New York: Norton.

Stamm, B. H. (Ed.). (1996). *Secondary traumatic stress: Self-care issues for clinicians, researchers and educators*. Lutherville, MD: Sidran Press.

| Chapter 9 | **Career themes in the lives of trauma therapists** |
|---|---|

Thriving and diversifying

I think in leaving the agency when their direction changed from working with trauma to more working alongside parents and teaching parenting skills, it helped me know where I wanted to continue working. I've been very clear in the last few years that I have certain skills and I think my philosophy makes me a fairly good person to be working in that field [trauma].

I've also become interested in work that's been done with refugees and their traumatic experiences and the new life that keeps occurring. It is also going into it at a deeper level and at the same time, I'm aware that part of my work although not all of my work is a strong interest in my role as a trainer and getting people to think through and develop their critical thinking. In terms of other directions, I can build upon my training in psychodrama, in terms of training counsellors and community workers.'

*Rose, counsellor-participant, reflecting on recent changes made to her work, adapted from Pack (2010)*

## Introduction

As the quote from Rose, one of the counsellor-participants above illustrates, career diversification along with lifestyle changes became personally necessary during agency restructuring as well as being professionally a savvy move in terms of self-care. Consistent with this view, Pearlman and Saakvitne (1995) mention this refocusing on more of a variety of roles beyond casework and therapy as being important to ameliorating the impact of work in the sexual abuse therapy field. At some level the counsellor-participants also acknowledged this need for personal and professional diversification in terms of roles, lifestyles and belief systems. Rose, after she experienced redundancy from her long-term position and employment as a therapist, saw herself positively developing into other work areas and roles. This diversification was supportive of other changes in relation to her growing spirituality and personal interests for her life more broadly.

As discussed in the previous chapter on spirituality, the counsellor-participants embarked on a search for meaning that involved a journey towards looking to find the self and the journey to look beyond the self. These are related processes with one search informing the other. The erosion of trust and esteem of others, as well as disruptions to helping professionals' own sense of the world as a safe place (Cunningham, 2003; Sabin-Farrell and Turpin, 2003) inevitably had effects on the lifestyles of the counsellor-participants. These shifts in belief and world view necessitated a search for a harmonious life–work flow which has been identified as being connected to the experience of working intensively with trauma disclosures, and more specifically, with work involving interpersonal violence (Huffam, 1999; Moulden and Firestone, 2007).

As discussed in previous chapters when one's initial training is challenged by the day-to-day experience of working with sexual assault survivors, existing frameworks or foundations for practice can seem not to 'fit', and as a consequence practitioners may experience a sense of disjuncture out of which they can find themselves practising in unknown territory or 'liminal spaces' (Myerhoff, 1982). Within such transitional zones, a search for alternative theories and lifestyles is generated in an attempt to make meaning of experience.

Aligning with the vicarious traumatization framework (Pearlman and Saakvitne, 1995) out of their search for alternatives, new meaning becomes attached to experience. This challenge, and the search provoked by this process, sits at the interface between the personal and professional aspects of a counsellor's world view and experiences. Therapy itself represents a liminal zone of 'betwixt and between' in which personal dilemmas and experiences can be deliberated upon. Experimentation with new strategies and ways of being can be evolved and tested for relevance in personal therapy, peer review and clinical supervision in cycles of action and reflection.

Napier and Fook (2001) had earlier interviewed social workers about defining moments in their practice. They discovered that while involving participants in an extended reflection on their most difficult practice scenarios, the participants came to view these practice experiences more positively. In a similar way, a critical incident approach asks participants about practice experiences that were interpreted as difficult at the time and then allows perceptions of the work to be examined (Lewis, 2008). As I was interested in the impact of these experiences on trauma therapists' career trajectories and life course, the vicarious traumatization literature provided an entry point to this discussion. I hypothesized that the intensity of the emotional impact of working with sexual abuse disclosures over time would explain the development of strategies that served to protect practitioners from the nature of the work (Pack, 2010).

As outlined in Chapter 2, five main themes were identified from the interviews. First, the motivations of counsellors for entering the field were based in family and personal biographies of trauma. Second, experiences of successful personal therapy informed clinical experiences. The counsellor-participants actively developed their own strategies that continued to guide their therapeutic work with clients throughout their careers. Third, immersion in sexual abuse work in the early 1980s meant that the counsellor-participants were 'trailblazers' in the field, creating their own theories about sexual abuse recovery to assist clients effectively in the absence of established theory at that time. Fourth, once the participants were established as expert practitioners in the field, personal and professional beliefs and theories were refined by practice wisdom, peer and supervisor support, and personal therapy. In this process, personal beliefs changed as different things came to matter, such as quality of life, relationship and spirituality. Fifth, a movement into alternative lifestyles and careers occurred while the counsellor-participants practised in the field of sexual abuse therapy over a number of years. This chapter focuses on the lifestyle changes that occurred during the 5–30 years of practice (Pack, 2010).

I discovered that over the length of their careers, spanning some 5–30 years, these sexual abuse therapists developed strategies for understanding their clients' trauma by reflecting on their own healing from traumatic events as well as from their experiences of working with clients who had been sexually abused. These integrated insights were drawn upon as a resource to guide therapeutic processes and to assist in maintaining their own resilience and on-the-job effectiveness. This awareness enabled them to continue to practise with sexually abused clients and to cope with disclosures that were 'hard to hear' as they integrated experiences from their earlier careers and from personal therapy, as well as insights from practice. Maintaining a balance of interests and roles was important as this ensured that the counsellor-participants retained a fresh perspective on themselves and their work. Diversifying into a range of work roles was increasingly appealing and realistic, including the development of a private practice. In a politically sensitive climate of public-funded trauma therapy covering some clients and not others, a portfolio of sub-specialties served as professional insurance in the face of changing fortunes. Bronwyn, one of the therapist consultants interviewed, for example, discussed the need to pace herself and to limit the number of new clients, particularly referrals for individual therapy to her private practice:

> Bronwyn: People invited me to take roles or be on committees or be in advisory groups or whatever. I was flattered into accepting because it sounded interesting and I was pleased to be chosen. That's the part I regret about not doing a bit more selecting – about what I could manage.

## Initial motivations: a call to service?

The counsellor-participants had worked in a range of occupations prior to entering the field of counselling and psychotherapy. Three had trained as ministers of religion before becoming trauma therapists. I wondered if this career development was influenced by the spiritual searching that went hand in hand with trauma work was itself a kind of spiritual journey embarked upon routinely.

Other occupations given by the counsellor-participants included cook, talkback host, soldier, clerk, bus driver, ambassador/public relations consultant, nurse, accountant, teacher/adult educator and secretary. With additional training, the group had become social workers, counsellors, psychologists and psychotherapists, reflecting the composition of the professions registered as trauma counsellors in New Zealand. Only three of the participants were men, reflecting the predominance of female therapists in the ACC's Register of Approved Counsellors, which forms the largest register of trauma-related specialist therapists in New Zealand.

As I have previously noted in prior chapters, once trained, the professional divisions among the counsellor-participants seemed less relevant as working in the field of sexual abuse/trauma established a connection among colleagues. I will therefore use the terms 'counsellor' and 'therapist' interchangeably, as these terms are the generic categories for the groups working with sexual abuse survivors. A common scenario was for a social worker, general counsellor or psychologist to train subsequently to become a psychotherapist. Therefore, it seemed artificial to impose one professional label when membership in more than one professional grouping applied. To illustrate the career diversification, we look first at Jill's career trajectory.

## Case study

### Jill's story

Jill, one of the counsellor-participants, initially trained as a social worker, later moving into training as a psychotherapist specializing in sexual abuse therapy. She balanced her therapy work with part-time hours teaching a bachelor of counselling degree at a local polytechnic. Her leisure interests included a range of artistic pursuits and storytelling as performance at a local theatre. The stories she told involved life themes of what a woman of her era was socially expected to do – become a mother early and take a job at a local bank 'because that is what good girls do' (Jill, personal communication). In among this social commentary were reflections of her own life, her feminist ideology and rights-based approach after witnessing many abuse narratives as a therapist with abuse survivors. In her personal life she had recently married her partner. She told me she had recently made friends with a group through her involvement in storytelling and creative arts that were sustaining and where she felt 'understood'. This balance of work, connection with like-minded others and other interests was useful as it meant she had options for achieving a quality of life that hitherto she had considered had been unavailable to her. She reflected that she could finally attain a lifestyle she had always dreamt about which involved establishing a private practice enabling a move to the country to live with her partner. In the small, rural community to which she moved, she soon became known for her work as a trauma therapist and had many clients contacting her for appointments through word of mouth and upon the recommendation of the local general practitioners in her area. Her partner found the initial phone calls from clients were interrupting their quality of life as Jill spent many hours on the phone with clients before they even made the initial appointment. It was his hope that Jill could eventually do less therapy and focus more on her artistic pursuits in the studio she had established. He also hoped that a move to a rural location could enable them both to improve their fitness by walks in the countryside as well as promoting an environment in which they could both find more time to rest and take 'time out' as they were both approaching retirement.

### Reflections on Jill's story

Finding a balance of roles and activities in everyday life is recommended in the vicarious traumatization literature, which also suggests that involvement in creative pursuits is important (O'Halloran and Linton, 2000). Maintaining relationships with family members is also deemed critical for maintaining wellness as we have seen in Chapter 4. In summary, Jill's narrative connects with the six domains defined as being critical to self-care that include the social, emotional, cognitive, physical, spiritual and vocational aspects that ideally need to be integrated as a whole lifestyle (O'Halloran and Linton, 2000).

Professor Lynne Jacobs, an academic, gestalt therapist and psychoanalyst, when asked about how she maintained her own self-care in her work as a therapist over many years at a roundtable discussion, had sage advice for the audience. Her self-care advice to therapists involved reference to sustaining relationships, maintaining a diverse range of hobbies, including her passion for baseball, and educating and teaching others about the process of doing therapy (Jacobs, 2006).

In relation to a question from the facilitator of a roundtable about self-care, Professor Jacobs echoed Jill's story about the need for balance and variety of activities, absorbing interests and involvement in intimate relationships in which one feels understood for the work one does as a trauma therapist. Like Jill, teaching was an important counterbalance to doing therapy:

> Jill: It's [self-care] about two things: one is the world of my intimate relationships. I realize how many of my friends are also therapists because these are people who can engage in a conversation about things that matter to me. [pause to reflect]
>
> Sports comes in there somewhere [audience laughs].

The other thing I realize is that actually doing things like these conferences – that is teaching and supervising and doing presentations, which is something I like to do when I am working as a therapist – I'm also learning things I will be able to teach with tomorrow. And I realize if I didn't have that in the structure of my life that I would probably burn out ...

(Jacobs, 2006)

## Later career progression

A theme for the counsellor-participants was a gradual progression into sexual abuse counselling. For the majority of those interviewed, after gaining some insight into the inadequacies of their existing work or lifestyle, in addition to some personal experience of trauma and recovery from trauma, different personal and career priorities emerged in their lives. Some had entered counselling and moved into managerial, supervisory and training roles. Four participants had published as a way of bringing their experience of particular issues they had encountered during their years of clinical practice into broader public awareness (Pack, 2010).

The participants' initial motivation for becoming trauma therapists was to heal some trauma in their own background or within their family of origin. Practitioners' motivation for entering the helping professions to address one's own experiences of trauma is a theme noted by other authors writing about trauma and resilience (Harms, 2015; O'Halloran and Linton, 2000). While self-care is seen as essential for clients, ironically this is a neglected field for the therapists who work with them (O'Halloran and Linton, 2000). The personal motivations to make a difference based on a sense of mission can, therefore, represent a political as well as personal agenda for involvement in the work of trauma recovery (Herman, 1992).

The shift from a focus on 'burnout' to 'secondary traumatic stress' (Stamm, 1996), 'vicarious traumatization' (Pearlman and Saakvitne, 1995) and 'compassion fatigue' (Figley, 1995) has intensified this responsibility for trauma therapists to 'heal thyself' in order to help others (O'Halloran and Linton, 2000). The professional codes of ethics also focus on self-responsibility for maintaining self-care practices that are conducive to remaining effective on the job.

Looking back on their careers with the advantage of hindsight, the counsellor-participants often recognized and acknowledged an unconscious motivation to work through some residual personal or family-of-origin issues that had not been dealt with previously. These included family issues in which the counsellor had played a helping role within their family of origin which was later professionalized; a variety of traumatic experiences that they had survived and which they now wished to assist others through; and the development and expression of various humanitarian and altruistic values. Hayley (her chosen pseudonym), one of the counsellor-participants, discussed the connections between her personal philosophy and her own personal experiences of trauma, and the ways in which these related to her decision to train as a social worker and, later, to become a sexual abuse counsellor:

Hayley: I think about wider social issues: about injustices between men and women there. I have strong feelings about equity and justice; that's why I work in the field that I do. And I think that this inequality is reflected in a nuclear family as well. So I think that people's histories have a huge impact on why things happen ...

So for me, too, like, my individual experience of abuse early on, I'm sure, is one of the reasons for getting into the area. I have been involved in this sense. As well I feel that people have a higher chance of resolving issues for themselves if they have the right kind of input. So I guess I have greater faith in people's abilities to change and develop if they are enthusiastic about being part of the counselling process. That involvement in counselling others has been a good thing for me.

## Family and personal experiences

The counsellor-participants who specialized as therapists in middle age often felt a sense of calling or mission as they matured in their professional experiences. Awareness of culture was an important factor in determining a lineage of healing within one's extended family narrative. Recently Harms (2015) writes of the importance of understanding trauma as involving a systemic approach beyond an individual focus for theorizing about the impact of trauma and the resilience that can develop in rebounding from traumatic experiences. Her example of Aboriginal Australians healing from intergenerational trauma is one example of this new direction in trauma theory from the Australian context (Harms, 2015). An intersubjective approach acknowledges the site of therapy as a co-created site. In a parallel sense vicarious traumatization also occurs in a co-created sense within the systems that surround the individual personal relationships and family, including extended family (Rasmussen, 2005).

For the two self-identified Māori counsellor-participants interviewed, the role of being a trauma therapist was one that their *whānau* had seen them assuming, as they were part of a lineage of healers. The strength drawn from this prophecy and the presence of ancestors within *whānau* [extended family], *hapū* [sub-tribe] and *iwi* [tribe] sharpened their resolve to pursue a career in one of the healing professions. Becoming a counsellor was seen by *whānau*, and by the individuals interviewed, as the fulfilment of a prophecy for their lives. Key moments were described as being pivotal to making this transition from the previous occupations of accountant and business woman to counselling and psychotherapy.

Maxine had made the transition from the profession of accountancy as a successful businesswoman to psychology after her grandmother's funeral and reading Māori creative writing, including the novel *Tangi* by Whiti Ihimaera (1989). This novel written by a Pacific poet and novelist, and the creative writing course Maxine was enrolled in, put her in touch with the presence of her grandmother now in spirit, who had prophesied her entry into the healing professions to carry on a family tradition of involvement in healing others. This prediction became a self-fulfilling prophecy as she then returned to university to study psychology:

> Maxine: My grandmother was a healer comfortable with spirituality. She would have been called a *matakite* [healer]. So, for me, it [counselling] was normal. She told my mother in Māori, because she didn't speak English, what I would be doing when I was eight years old. Of course, resistance was my forte; my first profession was accountancy until I returned to high school and studied Māori poetry (*Tangi* and the poetry of Hone Tūwhare). And my direction changed completely. Spirituality is one of the only reasons I would do this work. Rather than a profession, it was a calling directed by my elders.
>
> (Pack, 2010)

In contrast, other counsellor-participants described their involvement in sexual abuse work as happening more by accident than by choice. However, on closer reflection, this progression was related to a barely realized acknowledgement that there were personal issues acting as a motivating force for entering the work – and for staying in it. Often, the counsellor-participants also had social connections with those already working in the sexual abuse field. Thus, they were well positioned to hear about job vacancies. In this excerpt from an interview, Rebecca spoke of a series of fortuitous coincidences that led her into a full-time position in a sexual abuse agency. She had already worked in this agency as a student while completing her clinical psychology training:

> Rebecca: I saw doing psychology as a way out of sexual abuse work. No, it [move-ment into sexual abuse work] wasn't a choice at all. It was just through my course; I had a placement. I went and did a little bit of voluntary work at the sexual abuse agency because I knew some of the people there and I needed a bit of money. Things fell together at the time they set up their programme and here they were looking for staff and here I was looking for a job. And it happened and it fitted my placement, the placement criteria, and I just decided to do it and I stayed. If I had seen the job in the newspaper then I wouldn't have applied.

## Formative experiences

Early expectations of the work usually failed to meet the day-to-day realities of it. Few felt adequately prepared for the situations they were confronted with on the job.

A common theme for the therapists finding themselves immersed in trauma therapy was doing one's best with the available knowledge base. Those who had management respon-sibilities in addition to doing therapy meant that the learning curve was particularly steep. Bronwyn, a consultant therapist, had started early in the profession and had been quickly promoted to positions of authority early in her career. This career trajectory had been chal-lenging of her emerging abilities:

> Bronwyn: Yes – I think I have had quite a full experience, and that's partly because I keep being either thrown into or diving into the deep end myself. I mean, for example, there I was at age thirty being appointed director of a national counselling agency with-out any counselling background initially, and so that was a mountain learning curve in a sense. I mean suddenly I was both responsible for an agency and learning to be a coun-sellor myself, and having just finished a degree and going through a marital break-up.

As previously discussed in the preceding chapters, working in the sexual abuse field in the early 1980s was experimental, both in New Zealand and internationally. The publication *The Courage to Heal* (Bass and Davis, 1988) quickly reached New Zealand and the focus group members and counselling advisors confirmed that it was heralded as one of the main self-help guides referred to by clients and counsellors in New Zealand (Huffam, 1999).

Working in the absence of established systems, knowledge and protocols hampered the counsellor-participants' efforts to provide what they considered to be effective and appro-priate services. They also described the backlash encountered from the public over their involvement in bringing abuse to wider attention. This backlash mirrored the subsequent litigation and legal proceedings that Bass and Davis themselves encountered in the United States following publication of *The Courage to Heal*. Later, such publications were brought into the 'false memory' debate and criticized for encouraging disclosure prior to adequate skill-building (Briere, 1996; Herman, 1992).

The gap between initial expectations, learned theory and practice-based experiences fuelled a search for alternative responses to working within agency structures. Sally, one of the counsellor-participants, described this critical-reflective process as guiding her own practice as an addiction counsellor within a female prison. A process of deconstruction and reconstruction assisted her in dealing with her own sense of being 'overwhelmed' by the people she encountered who had been abused. Beth, one of the counsellor-participants, was led to specialize as a trauma counsellor in order to respond to a need her clients had identified. This enabled her clients to have access to a service they could afford as it was publically fully funded or subsidised:

> Beth: I absolutely didn't ever sit down and say to myself that I wanted to become a sexual abuse counsellor and head in that direction. It certainly wasn't like that. I moved from being in adult education to become a counsellor because I wanted to have both lots of skills and one led to the other. Within the first few months of being a counsellor I had requests from clients saying they wanted to do sexual abuse work and I was able to do it with them, as I was ACC registered. And so in the course of clinical supervision, I realised that sexual abuse work didn't have to be a foreign category: it was a logical extension of working with grief and self-esteem.

## The move to private practice

Over the time that they had been registered as trauma therapists, many of the counsellor-participants had, for a variety of reasons, moved from working in an agency to working in private practice. For some, this movement was seen as a way of resolving conflicts with agency politics and protocols, by either establishing a private practice or entering a group private practice with colleagues. Group practices were helpful for developing a shared ethos and for organizing the workplace administratively to suit those working together. Having greater control over the way in which the workplace was organized was considered important.

Another background theme behind the movement to private practice was the rapid change that was occurring in the helping professions in New Zealand during the 1990s, which has continued into 2016 with revisions to the ACC's contracting and funding protocols for trauma therapy. Workplace change, including widespread restructuring and re-organization within the public, charitable and voluntary helping sectors, meant that two of the counsellors interviewed had been made redundant from their employing agencies after 10–15 years of service, due to the changing focus of the agency. Both individuals were in the process of finding other work, which included some component of private practice. Having greater flexibility for organizing work systems and having greater control over the work setting were among the motivations behind the move into private practice. This movement into private practice as a result of disillusionment with agency work following restructuring has been discussed in the research literature (van Heugten, 1999) in order to account for the movement of social workers into private practice in New Zealand. For the counsellor-participants, this movement into private work may also reflect the nature of their specialization in the sexual abuse/trauma fields. Due to the public availability of funding directly to providers registered to undertake sexual abuse therapy with clients who had sexual abuse claims, this specialization seemed to lend itself to private work.

## Intergenerational patterns

The intergenerational patterns of abuse that the counsellor-participants witnessed day by day suggested that societal factors were often discussed as a significant background factor in sexual abuse. The writings of theorists who combined this kind of sociopolitical or structural analysis were among the resources the counsellor-participants found to be the most useful to draw upon. Awareness of sexual abuse as a prevalent phenomenon, particularly for women and children, came as an uncomfortable realization for some of the counsellor-participants. In this context, they discussed a growing awareness that those in their social networks, close friends or family members had been either victims or perpetrators of abuse. This realization brought with it a more personal awareness of the effects and repercussions of abuse. It was difficult to separate these more personal experiences from the day-to-day work, and inevitably they had an impact on the counsellors' routine functioning.

In small rural communities, awareness of the identities of victims and/or perpetrators increased. Supervision support from those not involved in the immediate situation was of assistance in dealing with such scenarios. Once abuse within a counsellor-participant's social network was disclosed, particular flashpoints of stress often began to affect the counsellor's general health and well-being. Learning to live with this knowledge, while challenging, enabled one of the counsellor-participants and her partner to emerge with strategies for dealing with abuse that was 'close to home':

> Rebecca: In fact, I think I have less impact [from the work]; no, that's not true. There's not less impact. I am less bothered by it now than I have ever been. I have had this personal stuff as well. Family members disclosed abuse within the family and I was abused. So there has been lots of fallout from that. And now the next bit of fallout will be what is life going to be for the next generation?

### Questions for reflection

- Reading about the counsellor-participants' lifestyles and the underlying motivations for making changes, are there any personal experiences of abuse that you have been coming to terms within your family of origin?
- What have the implications been of learning about these intergenerational patterns?
- What more do you need to do in terms of personal therapy and changing lifestyles to bring greater harmony in your personal/professional life?
- List three goals you have about the lifestyle you are aspiring to create currently or in the future.

## Personal experience of trauma

Many of the counsellor-participants interviewed described some early or formative experiences of trauma as children, including sexual and physical abuse. This theme is similarly reflected in the literature of helping professionals disclosing traumatic personal histories (Follette *et al.*, 1994; Martin *et al.*, 1986; Pope and Feldman-Summers, 1992). When facilitating therapy with clients, the counsellor-participants described drawing on a vast pool of intuitive wisdom and knowledge to guide their work. I often heard from those who were survivors that they could not envisage knowing how to guide therapeutic processes were it not for this knowledge. Their experiential insights, arising from their own knowledge, were often described as being more important than any of the conventional theories propounded in psychology textbooks.

The counsellor-participants also used this knowledge to engage in social and political action to address the societal myths about abuse and to work actively towards greater social equity. Balancing work in the therapy field with working towards social change has been recommended as an antidote to vicarious traumatization (Pearlman and Saakvitne, 1995). The counsellor-participants concurred with this recommendation. Therapists' personal experiences of sexual abuse or other trauma seemed to sharpen their resolve to pursue political action promoting social change. For Hayley, counselling survivors was seen as a natural outworking of her values and personal philosophy:

> Hayley: In terms of the trauma work, I would say, the personal experience was one of the pieces and the positive experience I had in terms of receiving counselling. If I go back even further to think of why I was so much into the rights issue, then it would be, as well, living in different cultures and seeing at a young age people who had a lot more rights than other people, yet who were able to affirm their rights less than other people. So that has always been there for me in terms of rights and justice issues.

## Consolidation and diversification

Pearlman and Saakvitne (1995) mentioned the need to diversify into a variety of roles as being important to ameliorating the impact of work in the sexual abuse field as therapists progressed in their careers. Diversification of roles was also seen by the counsellor-participants as important to remain 'fresh' in their practice.

Sometimes changing the balance of one's work was enough to restore the harmony in one's life and to remain professionally effective. Several of the counsellor-participants had made a decision to do less work in the trauma field and had commenced a plan for moving to the country to start a private practice in a rural location, combined with agricultural/horticultural projects.

Building houses, establishing gardens and lifestyle farms, and establishing businesses from home were part of what was considered to be 'the good life'. There was a desire for greater economic self-sufficiency based in spiritual philosophies and planning for retirement. Improving the quality of life was encompassed in Sally and her husband's vision for their joint future together which combined his insurance business, Sally's therapy practice and flower-growing for the florist industry from their home:

> Sally: I always like to keep a bit of a mix as a retirement project. We were talking just yesterday because we had a financial advisor at home yesterday talking about the flowers and my husband said: 'in about two to three years' time I would like to retire completely but your work is such that if you want to continue, you can. And we will have a very pleasant balance'. It sounded great! [laughs]

In practice, the counsellor-participants said it was difficult to reduce or change workloads, as they had gained a 'niche' by specializing in particular kinds of work. The combined pressures of their commitment to clients and difficulties with securing continuing funding for therapy informed their decision to reduce work or leave the field completely for a new start. This theme concurs with Devilly *et al.*, (2009) findings that beliefs about one's safety (an aspect that is included in the original vicarious traumatization framework), including in this definition organizational factors, combine to contribute to therapist distress.

## An awareness of dissonance

Coming through periods of stress and fatigue often suggested the need for longer-term solutions to address counsellor-participants' stress and trauma. I have conceptualized the periods in which counsellors experienced stress evoked by the nature of sexual abuse counselling as 'dissonance' as they grappled with the gap between the known and the unknown. This 'between' place fits with the idea that counsellors dealing with trauma operate in a transitional zone where they actively make meaning of experience. Etherington (2000), for example, described her experience of existing in a 'liminal zone' in experiencing vicarious traumatization when researching sexual abuse survivors' personal narratives. She concluded that supervision needs to attend to the supervisee's strategies for self-care. Echoing the counsellor-participants' experiences, she recommended 'a conscious positioning of self' to attach meaning to experience (Etherington, 2000: 387).

As we have seen in previous chapters in theorizing from past research with trauma therapists, this dissonance occurs when one's initial training and knowledge lack a sense of fit with the requirements of the job or practice setting, or when existing skills and knowledge are applied to a new field of practice, or when organizational reporting is required in particular formats and time frames that are incongruent with maintaining a relational stance with clients. Such dissonance can itself be a condition of working with sexual abuse and other traumatic disclosures, in terms of the potential for vicarious traumatization and burnout that are routinely experienced in trauma-related work (Pearlman, 1997; Pearlman and MacIan, 1995).

## Conclusion

Through a sustained reflection on their own experiences and a structural analysis of their own personal and wider socio-economic oppressions, the counsellor-participants were brought into contact with a sense of dissonance in themselves and their practice. In liminal spaces, they integrated practice wisdom into their scheme of knowing. Through this process, the counsellor-participants found it easier to put their exposure to traumatic events into a framework that accounted for what had happened to them and their clients, and to place it within a broader sociocultural paradigm. Contact with traumatic material, paradoxically, enabled them to move on with their own lives with a deeper awareness. This awareness was related to a number of variables.

Coming to terms with one's own experiences of abuse and trauma, along with a realization of intergenerational family patterns, challenged existing belief systems. The counsellor-participants' experiences of personal therapy offered a way of understanding and managing their over-identification with clients' trauma and their own countertransferential responses. With adjustments to work and the workplace by way of a move to private practice and project work, the counsellor-participants felt they had more choices about the ways in which they worked. By restoring a better life–work balance through movement to rural locations and diversification into new roles, new options for a fulfilling, self-sustaining future became available.

By integrating these learnings holistically in their personal and professional lives through peer support, clinical supervision and working towards greater work–life balance, the stresses of the work were currently seen as more episodic than continuous, in contrast to the way they had experienced these sources of stress earlier in their careers.

## Closing thoughts: Bronwyn's advice about maintaining balance

Bronwyn: Another phenomenon that occurs to trauma therapists over time is that at first it's so fascinating, at first it feels such a privilege, at first it's such an adventure in terms of being in touch with survivors personally in ways that you never expected. But if you do it for too long, for too much, too much of it every day then that fatigue factor wears in, which is why I'm really pleased to have cut my practice back to a more manageable level. With recent changes made I feel more attentive and more alert again than I've done in years.

## Taking stock of your current lifestyle and work–life balance

Thinking about Bronwyn's advice above, is your current caseload and work–life balance about right? If not consider the following points in making adjustments:

- Think back on a time when things were working well for you. If not in the present then reflect on a period in your recent past.
- What was different about this time in terms of your health, housing, nutrition, exercise, spiritual connection, intimacy in relationships, daily activities and work–leisure balance?
- How did you feel?
- How could you create/recreate some of the positive aspects of your lifestyle at that time?
- What do you need to do more of in your current lifestyle?
- What do you need to do less of?
- How can you inspire the hope that originally led you to train as a trauma therapist?
- List three goals for rebalancing your current lifestyle, caseload mix and work–life balance. You might wish to time-frame these goals and break larger goals into manageable steps if they are very broad, long-term goals. For example, moving home and family to a rural lifestyle from an urban one, or diversifying your current balance of work from 100 per cent therapy to a mix of other activities such as teaching, political lobbying/action for social change, research and supervision, may be a starting point to thinking about which areas require adjustment.

Jot down three initial thoughts as to where you wish to start to make changes to your current lifestyle.

## References

Bass, E. and Davis, L. (1988). *The courage to heal: A guide for women survivors of child sexual abuse*. New York: Perennial.

Briere, J. (1996). *Therapy for adults molested as children: Beyond survival* (2nd edn, revised and expanded). New York: Springer.

Cunningham, M. (2003). Impact of trauma work on social work clinicians: Empirical findings. *Social Work*, *48* (4), 451–9.

Devilly, G., Wright, R. and Varker, T. (2009). Vicarious trauma, secondary traumatic stress or simply burnout? Effect of trauma therapy on mental health professionals. *Australian and New Zealand Journal of Psychiatry*, *43* (4), 373–85.

Etherington, K. (2000). Supervising counsellors who work with survivors of childhood sexual abuse. *Counselling Psychology Quarterly*, *13* (4), 377–89.

Figley, C. R. (1995). *Compassion fatigue*. New York: Brunner/Mazel.

Follette, V. M., Polusny, M. and Milbeck, K. (1994). Mental health and law enforcement professionals: Trauma history, psychological symptoms, and the impact of providing services to child sexual abuse survivors. *Professional Psychology: Research and Practice*, *25* (3), 275–82.

Harms, L. (2015). *Understanding trauma and resilience*. London: Palgrave Macmillan.

Herman, J. (1992). *Trauma and recovery*. New York: Basic Books.

Huffam, L. F. (1999). A balancing act: Therapists' experience of working with sexual offenders (unpublished master's thesis). Wellington: Victoria University of Wellington.

Ihimaera, W. (1989). *Tangi*. Auckland: Heinemann Reed.

Jacobs, L. (2006). Round table discussion, GANZ Conference, Melbourne.

Lewis, I. (2008). With feeling: Writing emotion into counselling and psychotherapy research. *Counselling and Psychotherapy Research*, *8* (1), 63–70.

Martin, C. A., McKean, H. E. and Veltkamp, L. J. (1986). Post traumatic stress disorder in police working with victims: A pilot study. *Journal of Police Science and Administration*, *14* (2), 98–101.

Moulden, H. M. and Firestone, P. (2007). Vicarious traumatization: The impact on therapists who work with sexual offenders. *Trauma, Violence and Abuse*, *8* (1), 67–83.

Myerhoff, B. G. (1982). *Number our days: Triumph of continuity and culture among Jewish old people in an urban ghetto*. New York: Simon & Schuster/Touchstone.

Napier, L. and Fook, J. (Eds). (2001). *Breakthroughs in practice: Theorising critical moments in social work*. London: Whiting & Birch.

O'Halloran, T. M. and Linton, J. M. (2000). Stress on the job: Self-care resources for counselors. *Journal of Mental Health Counseling*, *22* (4), 354–65.

Pack, M. (2010). Career themes in the lives of sexual abuse counsellors. *New Zealand Journal of Counselling*, *30* (2), 75–92.

Pearlman, L. A. (1997). Trauma and the self: A theoretical and clinical perspective. *Journal of Emotional Abuse*, *1* (1), 7–25.

Pearlman, L. A. and MacIan, P. S. (1995). Vicarious traumatization: An empirical study of the effects of trauma work on trauma therapists. *Professional Psychology: Research and Practice*, *26* (6), 558–65.

Pearlman, L. A. and Saakvitne, K. W. (1995). *Trauma and the therapist: Countertransference and vicarious traumatization in psychotherapy with incest survivors*. New York: W. W. Norton.

Pope, K. S. and Feldman-Summers, S. (1992). National survey of psychologists' sexual and physical abuse history and their evaluation of training and competence in these areas. *Professional Psychology: Research and Practice*, *23* (5), 353–61.

Rasmussen, B. (2005). An intersubjective perspective on vicarious trauma and its impact on the clinical process. *Journal of Social Work Practice*, *19* (1), 19–30.

Sabin-Farrell, R. and Turpin, G. (2003). Vicarious traumatization: Implications for the mental health of health workers? *Clinical Psychology Review*, *23* (3), 449–80.

Stamm, B. H. (Ed.). (1996). *Secondary traumatics Stress: Self-care issues for clinicians, researchers and educators*. Lutherville, MD: Sidran Press.

van Heugten, K. (1999). Social workers who move into private practice: A study of the issues that arise for them (unpublished doctoral thesis). Christchurch, New Zealand: University of Canterbury.

# Chapter 10 **Conclusion and your self-care plan**

## Considerations and next steps

I think it should be mandatory that therapists do their own work [personal therapy], because it keeps you in touch with the process. I think you can get into a bit of a holier-than-thou situation if you are always in the therapist's chair, so it helps to feel that vulnerability from time to time. I think you get choosier about therapists and most of us are doing some sorts of training as well. I'm a bit of a personal growth junkie [laugh].

*Sophia, counsellor-participant talking about her learning in personal therapy as a source of personal development for her role as a therapist*

## Introduction

In this chapter, we draw together the themes presented throughout the nine chapters of this book and suggest how each comprises a dimension of a multilayered approach to self-care for trauma therapists. As we can see over the past 30 years in the professional literature, there has been increasing interest in clinician self-care and the effects of working continually with traumatic disclosures over many years. In the past decade, there has been a shift from generic stress and burnout to the impact of the work on trauma professionals in terms of the specific challenges they face in working with traumatized populations of clients. The codes of ethics of many psychology, counselling and psychotherapy professional associations now incorporate standards of practice and ethical values that place responsibility on practitioners to seek appropriate support and consultation to maintain our own health and well-being as trauma therapists. The challenge for therapists is to care for oneself when one's training may have been focused on ensuring the therapeutic outcomes for the client (O'Halloran and Linton, 2000). As much psychotherapy and helping professional training is designed to ensure the well-being of the client appropriately, there is the tendency for therapist education and ongoing professional development to overlook the emotional and psychological needs and requirements of the therapist and the relationship of therapist well-being to good therapeutic process and outcomes (O'Halloran and Linton, 2000). This book was written in the hope of addressing some of the main issues for therapists engaged in hearing traumatic disclosures daily on the job. The ideas are not meant to be prescriptive but are based in my research over the past 15 years with trauma therapists and include my own reflections as a practitioner. The intention of this book is to join the dialogue to add to the increasing body of knowledge about therapist self-care. This knowledge base includes a variety of publications such as professional journal articles, conferences and research that are focused on theorizing about protective practices and their relationship to trauma therapists' well-being.

## Dimensions of therapist self-care

There are several areas of self-care that are important to attend to when routinely dealing with traumatic material with one's clients on the job. Many of these aspects are interrelated. These dimensions include dealing with one's own personal experience of trauma while witnessing the trauma of others; learning how to witness the pain of trauma survivors safely; and actively authoring and re-authoring one's personal/professional narratives and ways of being that ameliorate the impact of the work. Finding a synthesis of theoretical frameworks for one's practice is also important. From the counsellor-participants' perspectives, the advice is to explore 'what works' and to incorporate a range of theoretical approaches, including but not limited to anti-oppressive, strengths-based and trauma-informed theory. This rich tapestry of theoretical approaches is also part of therapist self-care, as it supports a more collaborative relationship with clients, thus buffering the sense of disjuncture that can occur when more 'top-down' relationships are engaged with therapeutically. The blank screen of Freudian psychoanalysis is now thought more generally to be unhelpful when working with trauma survivors as there is potential for retriggering issues with past figures when skill-building is needed prior to memory work to approach the processing of traumatic memory safely (Herman, 1992, 2010). Therefore, knowledge of relational, psychodynamic and narrative theories of practice are all essential in the repertoire of trauma therapists' clinical training. Working within such theories positions therapists more collaboratively with clients that the counsellor-participants found supportive of their own resilience as their ethical practices aligned with their personal philosophies more fully when such frameworks of practice were worked within (Pack, 2010a).

Career and lifestyle diversification, addressing workplace/team culture and ensuring preventive and supportive strategies such as clinical supervision and comprehensive CISM are all important aspects of self-care. For those who move into private and group practices, networking to maintain engagement in collegial relationship within a community of peers is also important. Awareness of self is the starting point, hence the mindfulness and spirituality practices detailed in Chapter 8 are central to determining what specific self-care strategies are needed by individual trauma therapists based on existing ways of being, belief systems and cultural backgrounds. Assessing one's own existing sources of sustenance is a useful place to start in developing a greater awareness of personal resources and needs. The healing potential of relationship is another area impacted by vicarious traumatization, therefore, awareness of therapist needs in terms of relationship requires ongoing attention (Pack, 2010b).

In Chapter 1, the terms vicarious traumatization, secondary traumatic stress and compassion fatigue were defined and the potential impact on the therapist outlined, with reference to the research literature. Second, I reviewed recent applications of the vicarious traumatization framework to suggest the way forward for the self-care of those working with survivors of trauma and sexual violence, drawing upon the concept of resilience. Third, drawing from ecological systems theory, I suggested a systemic model of vicarious traumatization, the experience of which I see as existing on several levels, with each impacting upon the next in a compounding or spiralling fashion (Pack, 2013, 2014). Attention to the diverse contexts in which therapists practise is also needed. Therefore, a systemic approach to therapist self-care on four different levels is needed. These levels I conceptualize as relating to the self of the therapist and immediate relationships with significant others; the therapeutic relationship between client and therapist; the interface between the therapist and the employing organization; and the societal discourses that surround the work of therapy for survivors of trauma and sexual violence (Pack, 2013, 2014).

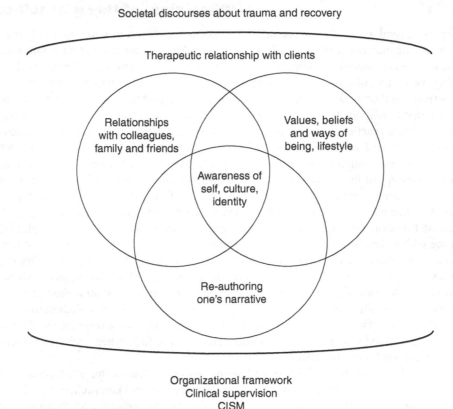

**FIGURE 10.1** Aspects of self-care

Figure 10.1 summarizes the different aspects of self-care discussed throughout this book.

In this concluding chapter, I will provide an illustration of how I see the dimensions of self-care working dynamically on each of the four levels mentioned above to propose interventions to address vicarious traumatization on each level. The implications for the self-care of those who provide counselling and therapeutic services to survivors of trauma are then discussed.

Before moving to consider the multidimensional model of self-care, the changing context of the field of trauma recovery, including the cultural dimensions of the impact of colonization in Australasia, first needs attention. So let's pause to reflect on and recap what some of those changes have been.

## Recent developments in trauma therapy in Australasia

Since moving to Australia to work and live in 2011, I have been refining my insights based in my original research with ACC-registered trauma therapists in New Zealand (Pack, 2004, 2009, 2010a, 2010b, 2012, 2013, 2014). In 2015 in Australia, a National Commission into Institutional Responses to Child Sexual Abuse was created, highlighting the needs of survivor clients, and the government's role and responsibility in the statutory provision of services for adult survivors of sexual violence who were abused as children in institutional care. Recently, I was asked to chair a public forum where representatives of the Roman Catholic church and the Salvation Army who were involved in services aimed to make compensation to victims, talked of their experiences. During one of the panel addresses, a 60-year-old, white Australian man who had witnessed and spoken up about abuse in his workplace, gave a poignant account of his early career as a residential social worker. In front of that audience, he wept as he described the way in which he had not been able to stop vulnerable children from being abused in institutional care as a 22-year-old social worker, despite bringing what he had observed to the attention of his managers. It occurred to me that vicarious traumatization is experienced also when therapists and other helping professionals encounter abuse they witness and can neither address at the time nor prevent for the future despite their best efforts. The aftermath of their experience is lingering while the ongoing guilt that they were unable to intervene to stop the abuse that happens in institutions and in the wider society remains a source of distress and vicarious traumatization. Each event witnessed traumatizes in a compounding way throughout a career with the internal dialogue: 'I should have been able to stop or prevent what happened' and even: 'I was complicit in the act'. Direct traumatization experiences can occur when practitioners' accounts are not heard and where there is denial about what is happening in the workplace or institution. Alternatively, there may be threats to career progression and advancement for those who speak up about what they see from those in positions of authority.

The Royal Commission into Institutional Responses to Child Sexual Abuse in Australia (www.childabuseroyalcommission.gov.au) brings such issues into sharp relief for helping practitioners and those who witness the abuse of children by others in their workplaces. Narratives of professionals who did not speak up about what they had observed of abuse in care, as evidenced in the experience of survivor hearings in the commission's fora, once again raises questions about the demands on therapists engaged in trauma-related work and the wider injustice they have witnessed over the years from engagement with trauma survivors. Adding to this complexity is the colonial past of both Australia and New Zealand and the legacy this leaves in relation to our context for practice.

The experience of intergenerational trauma and abuse of Aboriginal and Torres Strait Islanders who lived through the enforced child removals as part of the Stolen Generation, is included in the National Commission's brief. As the agency in which sexual violence and trauma work takes place is itself informed by the societal values in which practice occurs, I argue that we need to be mindful of the societal discourses surrounding work in the sexual violence field and to integrate these understandings in our practice with survivors of sexual violence and trauma. The reformulated view of self-care, therefore, is to present and reflect on the implications of an ecological systems theory approach to vicarious traumatization and resilience, and to suggest why as practitioners we need to take systemic factors into account in the course of providing therapy for survivors of trauma. Connecting with like-minded colleagues for advocacy to address injustice witnessed during client disclosures is a starting point to a range of responses, including political action and activism.

## Recapping: themes from the vicarious traumatization and resilience literature

In my own research, the counsellor-participants suggested to me that vicarious traumatization was a temporary experience, more common in the first five years of practice, over which time refined and matured ways of being were actively developed and then were available to apply as protective factors (Pack, 2004, 2009, 2010a, 2010b, 2012). This finding aligns with studies on resilience which report more positive outcomes than originally predicted in the vicarious traumatization framework (McCann *et al.*, 2013; van Heugten, 2013). Personal growth and positive change arising from trauma-related engagement is reported in the experience of therapeutic work with survivors (Linley and Joseph, 2007). There is increasing confidence in asserting a place for contextual factors that apply to the study of vicarious traumatization to develop notions of resilience. The concept of resilience, based within the risk and resilience literature, focuses on how practitioners develop a range of protective factors to sustain them in their witnessing of their survivor clients' healing journey, as they constructively deal with the rigours of working with disclosures of sexual violence and trauma (Marcus and Dubi, 2006; Moran, 2002; van Heugten, 2013). Paradoxically, navigating the rigours of trauma-related work is thought necessary to develop positive ways of being, through an active engagement with the experience of vicarious traumatization to evolve these protective factors (Linley and Joseph, 2007; McCann *et al.*, 2013).

Becoming more aware of one's 'narrative identity' (White, 1995, 1997), including the goals and aspirations therapists have for their lives, is also a protective factor in rebounding from episodes of vicarious traumatization. I have suggested in Chapters 2 and 3 that re-authoring of the therapist's narrative identity (White, 1995, 1997) through a critical-reflective process is one of the buffering factors to vicarious traumatization. Chapters 5, 6 and 7 suggest that this re-authoring also needs to occur in the discourses surrounding the team, organization and supervisory relationships. Chapter 4 discussed the impact of the work on relationships, personal and professional, and Chapters 8 and 9 explored changes to world view and belief systems, both of which influence lifestyle, work–life balance and spirituality.

## How vicarious traumatization impacts

The severity or degree of impact of vicarious traumatization from engagement with sexual abuse trauma is thought to vary from worker to worker, based in variables such as personal biography, including past experiences of sexual violence and traumatic events; training and education; personality styles; and existing self-care strategies (Pack, 2013, 2014). Those areas of the therapist's life routinely impacted include the relationship between self and other, sense of safety and personal security, the capacity for intimacy and connection with others and sense of self-efficacy (Pearlman and Saakvitne, 1995). When therapists draw upon their own self-awareness, they are more available for encouraging survivor clients to find their own spiritual strength and purpose (Bloemhard, 2008). Therefore, therapists who work with survivors of trauma and sexual violence are also encouraged to embark on a parallel journey of recovery to their survivor clients. Vicarious traumatization can affect those professional and personal significant others who are in a close relationship with the counsellor as vicarious traumatization impacts upon the self of the counsellor. When vicarious traumatization is impacting, distancing from social contact and intimacy is a feature of the experience, leading to social isolation and withdrawal if unattended (Pearlman and Saakvitne, 1995).

## Factors promoting therapist resilience

Alongside the negative orientation of the vicarious traumatization literature, there is a burgeoning body of research on how clinicians manage actively the effects of engagement with traumatic disclosures from their clients. This research has highlighted that education and awareness of self as a routine experience is critical in the self-care of clinicians, enabling them to normalize their responses, to 'bounce back' and survive the rigours of trauma-related helping. Including self-awareness activities such as meditation and involvement in community, clinical supervision and personal therapy are all considered to be helpful for promoting therapists' resilience to stress and trauma (Canfield, 2005; Sommer, 2008).

Therapist resilience is a newer concept that represents a critique of the original vicarious traumatization framework (Collins and Long, 2003). Drawing from the risk and resilience literature, the concept of resilience suggests that individual clinicians actively evolve positive processes and strategies to maintain their therapeutic effectiveness when dealing with traumatic disclosures from their clients (Canfield, 2005; Collins and Long, 2003).

The presence of a range of protective factors is thought to be evolved in the face of vicarious traumatization and engagement with trauma (Collins and Long, 2003). These protective practices include the accessing and use of social and collegial supports; maintaining an attitude of 'optimistic perseverance' (Medeiros and Prochaska, 1998); humour; involvement in community to foster a sense of belonging/connection to others; sustaining hobbies and effective use of leisure time; spirituality; and involvement in political activity for improving social justice (Johnson and Hunter, 1997; McCann *et al.*, 2013; Marcus and Dubi, 2006; Moran, 2002). Developing a multi-theoretical framework for practice was another factor enabling the counsellor-participants to maintain a fresh perspective in their work with survivors (Pack, 2010a, 2014).

Being surrounded by people who understand the nature of trauma sexual abuse recovery work and its impact, I discovered in my research with trauma therapists that relationships with friends and family was another important aspect of resilience to enable therapists to rebound from experiences of vicarious traumatization (Pack, 2004, 2010b). This research encompassed a breadth of opinion about the relevance of the vicarious traumatization framework from 22 therapists across a range of professions, including social workers, clinical psychologists, counsellors and psychotherapists who were registered with the ACC to provide a specialized service to survivors of sexual violence (Pack, 2004, 2009, 2010a, 2010b).

In interviewing the counsellor-participants about the relevance of the vicarious traumatization framework, I had assumed that personal relationships would be very important to sustain therapists in the course of their work. What I discovered to my surprise was that the work had transformed the nature of these intimate and family relationships. Their marriages, partnerships and friendships changed over the course of involvement in sexual abuse and trauma recovery work with a movement towards the development of sustaining personal relationships with those who worked in the same field (Pack, 2010b). The movement to align personal with more professionally based relationships enabled the therapists to feel better understood by those whom they lived with, though these changes were painful and difficult to make in the short term (Pack, 2010b).

## How vicarious traumatization impacts in the workplace

Sexual abuse counsellors, social workers and therapists risk becoming secondarily and vicariously traumatized in their work with survivors of trauma due to the nature of traumatic work, which has been described as a 'contagion' if entered into without sufficient preparation and training (Herman, 1992). Some of the contextual factors about how trauma impacts on the worker lie in the organizational setting in which the therapy takes place. For example, the lack of adequate time and resources, such as clinical supervision, including time for reflection on one's own actions, can result in trauma and stress that can impact upon the client and worker compromising therapeutic gains and the healing process for the client (Canfield, 2005; Cunningham, 2003; Etherington, 2000, 2009).

In the New Zealand context, research studies have suggested that what is defined as 'stressful' includes the experience of direct traumatization through intimidation and experiences of horizontal violence by co-workers as well as oppressive systems of management (van Heugten, 2007, 2010). Media reports of systemic failures frequently are made against a backdrop of a culture of crisis management in which there is a lack of reflective space and time for training and supervision of the workers involved. Claims of 'harassment' and 'bullying' within the workers' employing organization are routinely reported in such contexts (McCann *et al.*, 2013; van Heugten, 2007, 2013).

In my own research with the counsellor-participants, I noted that there was a mismatch of philosophies that was a source of vicarious traumatization reflecting the different ethical and moral positioning of the therapists. Legal and medically based agencies who work with survivors often do so in crisis intervention mode where the primary effort is to enforce the law or provide medical treatment in order to restore the status quo as quickly as possible (Pack, 2013, 2014). This kind of environment coupled with 'top-down', non-consultative frameworks can stifle creativity and reflection. Within the context of multidisciplinary teams, those working with survivors of sexual violence sometimes report experiencing a sense of dissonance in the helping endeavour due to their differing approaches to practice and theoretical paradigms (Pack, 2004, 2009, 2012). Work with trauma survivors is congruent with strengths-based, emancipatory, narrative and social justice paradigms, prefaced on the notion that the professional works collaboratively with clients to focus on fostering autonomy and self-determination in the therapeutic process. If the structure of the agency does not foster this non-hierarchical consultative approach, workers can search for private practice options as alternative workplaces more consistent with the approach needed for practice (Pack, 2004, 2009, 2010b). The movement towards working with survivors of sexual violence in private practice settings through activities that enable new meaning-making from experience is a protective practice for trauma therapists facing such organizational dilemmas (Pearlman and Saakvitne, 1995). The trend of psychotherapists moving to private practice settings is one consequence of this dissatisfaction with more authoritarian management styles prevailing in employing organizations and contracting arrangements (van Heugten, 2007, 2010, 2013).

When organizations and teams focus on the individual client and ignore the wider sociopolitical context in which trauma and abuse occur, this residual focus tends to conflict with the workers' personal philosophies, and this highlights the dissonance between theory and practice (Pack, 2004, 2009, 2010b). If unaddressed, the effects of working with trauma can have wide-ranging implications for the organization as a whole (Sexton, 1999). Individual experiences of vicarious traumatization can have a destabilizing effect on the teams in which workers are vicariously traumatized, which in turn can have a ripple effect on interpersonal communication, effectiveness on the job and organizational functioning (Pack, 2004, 2012; Sexton, 1999). An example of how the organizational culture employing therapists to work with survivors of trauma and sexual violence can impact on the counsellor is illustrated by the policies and practices of the ACC of New Zealand. Since the ACC (the public funder of most trauma therapy in New Zealand) changed its focus to a business model in recent years with more frequent and detailed reporting requirements and the need to tender for service through an ACC-registered third-party manager, there has been a drop-out of some therapists doing this work and reductions in numbers of sensitive claims being accepted (Hayward,

2009). These media reports suggest that there are systemic issues at play in the contracting of therapists and acceptance of sensitive claims on which the eligibility for public funding for victims is based. This has led to collective action by ACC therapists to challenge the status quo (Hayward, 2009). Harms (2015) suggests the usefulness of a multi-theoretical, holistic and systemic view of recovery in the assessment and treatment of trauma survivors. A multi-theoretical and systemic approach to vicarious traumatization, including theorizing and working with trauma, is suggested in a parallel way that the treatment of victims is recommended in my own research with trauma therapists (Pack, 2014). This holistic, systemic approach to addressing vicarious traumatization has manifold implications for therapist self-care, which I will now turn to describe and explain.

## A systems approach to vicarious traumatization and therapist self-care

The conceptual framework that explains the importance of the support networks that surround the individual is best described within the ecological systems model of human development, pioneered by Bronfenbrenner (1994). This contextual view takes the perspective of the interventions needed on the levels of the micro- (relating to the individual), meso- (relationships between the individual and micro-systems), exo- (broader settings such as institutions and organizations) and macro-systems (relating to society as a whole and the discourses that surround it) to sustain and develop the individual from a human development perspective. Trauma therapists work at every point of interaction from the individual outwards to society at large by endeavouring to address the myths that surround interpersonal violence and abuse. The very same systems are a part of trauma therapists' self-care. The earlier research I have undertaken with ACC-registered therapists suggested that intervention is required within each system to create healthy workers within healthy workplaces to ameliorate vicarious traumatization on the individual level as well as to assist development of the sexual abuse and trauma therapy workforce as a whole (Pack, 2004, 2013, 2014). The benefits of these systems working well ultimately assisted the recovery process of survivors engaged in therapy (Pack, 2013).

These micro-systems applied to work with survivors of trauma and sexual violence involve interventions on four levels: the level of the individual counsellor's responses; the level of the therapeutic relationship between the client and therapist and the resources needed to sustain them in the work; the organizational level; and the level of the societal discourses surrounding trauma and sexual violence which influences the counselling profession as a whole. I will now turn to describe components on each level to illustrate the interdependence of each to the next which exist in a dynamic interplay.

- The micro-level: this level I have conceptualized as relating to the individual well-being of the therapist and client. This micro-system deals with therapists' own awareness of self in the practitioner role and how the work with survivors of sexual violence/trauma is impacting. On this level, resources are needed to address the impact of traumatic transference and countertransference, support for managing on-the-job stress, the availability of peer support, affirming personal and professional relationships and networks, and the availability of personal therapy.
- The meso-level: this level I have conceptualized as the interface between the therapist and the resources surrounding them to sustain them in the work. Resources needed to ameliorate vicarious traumatization on this level include training programmes and

mentoring and clinical supervision that deals with vicarious traumatization using relational and trauma-informed models such as those recommended by Etherington (2000, 2009) and Knight (2006). Integration of a range of theoretical models underpinning recovery is important to guide the therapist in the process of the work (Pack, 2010a).

- The exo-level (the organizational level): on this level I have conceptualized the culture of the agency as ameliorating or compounding vicarious traumatization. If the surrounding workplace culture normalizes vicarious traumatization by including a range of debriefing and peer support within day-to-day case meetings/teamwork and involving non-hierarchical collaborative decision-making, these factors working together can act as 'buffers' to vicarious traumatization. Having a culture that sees vicarious traumatization as a normal part of trauma-related helping in which dialogue is encouraged within case meetings about the effects of the work is essential to self-care on this level. This culture can provide a sense of security for the worker to freely discuss responses to the work without fear of censure or compromising promotional prospects (Sexton, 1999). Having a sense of 'collective ethics' (Reynolds, 2011), where therapists in group practices and teams describe to one another their differing understandings of how each therapist's personal ethical code relates to the collective effort which is enacted to guide their work, is critical. Such sharing of ethical dilemmas to externalize rather than internalize public issues such as sexual abuse trauma is an opportunity for acts of collective witnessing (Reynolds, 2011).

- The macro-level: on this level I have conceptualized support from the professional associations in terms of education about vicarious traumatization in programmes of ongoing professional development. Professional development may, for example, occur through the distribution of research findings, journal publication with vicarious traumatization special issues, and conferences focused on vicarious traumatization and developing resilience in the workforce as a whole (Pack, 2013, 2014).

Responses on the macro-level can suggest acts of advocacy and political activism in situations where there is structural inequality witnessed by therapists in their work. This can involve the poverty and the powerlessness and injustice trauma survivors suffer as a consequence of their experiences. Where therapists lack adequate or supportive work conditions and resourcing to address these issues, this collective witnessing of client pain that cannot be addressed by individual therapy alone (Reynolds, 2011). Attendance at professional conferences, webinars and workshops is one means of bringing therapists together to address these issues. Figure 10.2 depicts how I see these levels interrelating within an ecological systems approach.

I will now move to look at each level in terms of the recommended interventions in more detail. These layers are not discrete but exist in relation to one another with each influencing the next (Pack, 2013, 2014).

## The micro-level: individual interventions for self-care

On this level there are multiple themes. The first is countering isolation by drawing upon key relationships that have opportunities to share experiences arising from the work in the trauma and sexual violence field. This sharing of experience ideally is linked to information/education about burnout, compassion fatigue and vicarious traumatization.

Individual supervision is another theme that all the counsellor-participants valued and actively used to support their practice in the field of trauma therapy. Clinical or professional supervision needs to have a relational focus to avoid the shame of disclosing the impact

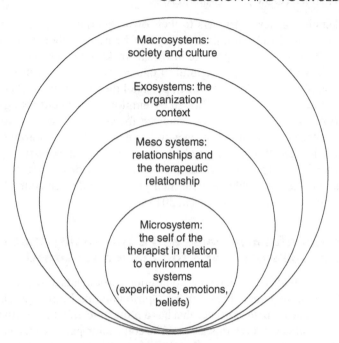

FIGURE **10.2** The ecological systems approach

of the work of trauma therapy (Harrison and Westwood, 2009). Clinical supervision may occur alongside peer networks or groups training workshops on anti-oppressive practice, to provide a means of ameliorating vicarious traumatization. Supervision may also act as a forum in which to discuss and learn from other therapists' strategies for self-care and serve as a reminder to implement these. Clinical supervision provides a forum to make changes to existing support strategies and lifestyles. Critical-reflective modes of supervision encourage therapists to actively review one's practice. More generally, the process of critical reflection is a means of debriefing workers from trauma and enables them to consider what they wish to do next time when faced by a similar situation in their practice. This self-critique of one's practice in retrospect, therefore, also enables trauma therapists to plan and self-monitor one's framework for practice both now and in the future (Napier and Fook, 2001).

Information on worker rights, through belonging to collectives and group practices with access to union representatives, may assist in supporting trauma therapists to individually as well as collectively advocate for conditions of employment that support their work. It is important that these areas of supervision and training are not superimposed with performance appraisal, however.

Finding creative ways of bringing one's personal and professional ethics into alignment with one's preferred way of being is a central focus for trauma therapists. Practising advocacy on behalf of disenfranchised or marginalized groups in society through political action is another consideration in preventing burnout and vicarious traumatization (Reynolds, 2011).

## The needs of survivor therapists

Personal therapy needs to be available to therapists who find that there are issues of their own abuse or trauma intruding into their day-to-day work. Personal therapy is one of the means by which workers encountering triggers to their own experience of abuse and oppression may use therapy to feedback insights and ways of being into their own emerging theories of practice. Critical-reflective practice in which workers engage in an ongoing analysis of themes in their work would seem helpful in tandem with personal therapy (Napier and Fook, 2001). Therefore, the linkages between personal therapy of the worker as a model for informing their practice needs to be affirmed by employers and contracting organizations. In the past, survivor therapists have been criticized for lacking objectivity to undertake the work and were asked by their funding agency to leave the field temporarily for the duration of their personal therapy. While this may be helpful for some therapists, my research suggests that survivor therapists who undertake their own therapy develop resources and insight that, over time, become a valuable basis for their practice, and these counsellors need to be appropriately supported in their work (Pack, 2013).

## Developing mindful awareness and a spirituality that is integrated in one's being as a foundation for practice

Mindfulness and spirituality facilitated the counsellor-participants to tolerate ambiguity and complexity while retaining hope (Pack, 2010a). Spirituality has been highlighted as a means of providing deeper meaning to existence that has a protective effect for victims and for therapists engaged in trauma work (Harms, 2015). The counsellor-participants who had left their churches as ministers of religion found that they begun to react to the patriarchal nature of the structures of organized religion. Exposure to abuse narratives from parishioners necessitated a reformulated spirituality, free from exploitation and the 'top-down' relationships. They said this reformulated, more egalitarian relationship with clients was essential to their continued practice as a trauma therapist (Pack, 2014).

Often mindfulness practices were integrated into everyday life. Such practices helped with awareness of self in daily life. What I have termed 'the search for self' involved various alternative and mind–body practices such as Reiki and Hakomi based in Eastern philosophies, and Vipassanā practices ranging from living in silence in remote places in nature, through to more conventional forms of personal therapy as personal development. Greater awareness of self and of being in the moment assisted the counsellor-participants to hold multiple perspectives and disturbing disclosures from clients, as these reformed spiritual understandings and lifestyles were ways of effectively processing traumatic material (Pack, 2013, 2014). This embodied awareness of self and physical surroundings has been noted in other research studies. Therapists involved in spirituality were found to develop a quality of presence when with the other and clarity crucial to the practice of empathy (Harrison and Westwood, 2009).

What I have called 'the search beyond self' involved ways in which the counsellor-participants found greater acceptance of self and other, patience and greater compassion for humanity. The boundaries between self and other were expanded, at the same time allowing an awareness of being out of balance with a need to engage in a withdrawal or consultation to gain perspective in the work with trauma survivors (Pack, 2013, 2014).

## Exo-levels: relationships with significant others

Changes to the world view of the therapist inevitably challenged the foundations of previous relationships. The transformation of the self was related to the development of a personal politics that aimed at social change. Intimate personal relationships for at least ten of the counsellor-participants changed over the duration of their careers spanning some 10–20 years. Longstanding marriages and partnerships broke up in favour of relationships that were more connected across the work lines (Pack, 2010b). Largely this is because the counsellor-participants who were working as trauma therapists had a need to feel understood which included an awareness of the pressures and experiences related to the nature of their work in the field of trauma. The counsellor-participants drew on understandings and ways of being that were at times quite different and at odds with the partners, adult children and friends who worked outside the trauma therapy field. They noted how the outlook of the therapists they lived with had been altered over time. They struggled to understand the therapists' revised frame of reference and belief system (Pack, 2010b). Where individuals and families lack access to reflective and liminal sites and like-minded others in which to explore and make meaning of their experience, there are implications for their ability to sustain relationships (Pack, 2013, 2014).

Taking stock of one's needs and whether the existing personal and intimate relationships are still sustaining are important for those involved in trauma therapy. This is an aspect of self-care to periodically review. Frank discussions are needed to explore what is also occurring for the significant others who are important in trauma therapists' lives, so that changes and adjustments in ways of relating can be openly explored to avoid a build-up of silent criticism and reprisals that can lead to unspoken hostility and distance in relationships (Pack, 2013, 2014).

## Dealing with personal histories of abuse within family

An awareness of abuse and trauma that has occurred within one's extended family and coming to a philosophical understanding about the prevalence of abuse and its effects were part of the experience of the counsellor-participants (Pack, 2013, 2014). This personal piece was particularly challenging when abuse was part of the family's history.

Part of the early years of practice involved sorting out what responses to stress and trauma belonged to the personal biography of the therapist. Second knowing how this early trauma experience can potentially affect the therapeutic relationship is important for therapists to become more aware and mindful of how the work is affecting them over time (Pack, 2013, 2014). For example, Pearlman *et al*. (1996: 35) acknowledge that:

> When a helper's ego resources are compromised, she is less likely to make decisions that are in her own best interest, and may make professional errors in boundaries, judgement or strategy. She may be less self-reflective and therefore unable to sort out her own feelings and responses from those of her clients. She may fail to set limits and may overextend herself, leading to inevitable failure, resentment and exhaustion. A psychotherapist will be less able to notice and then analyse and use her own countertransference, thus leaving the therapy vulnerable to countertransference enactments.

Holding appropriate limits and self–other boundaries were considered important dimensions of self-care by the counsellor-participants when dealing with one's own abuse issues as a therapist so that they are not unconsciously superimposed onto the client (Pack, 2013, 2014). Issues that brought therapy to an impasse in my own research with the counsellor-participants included the therapist's countertransference triggered by the client's characteristics or personality or the process of the therapeutic relationship in which dissociation of the therapist due to traumatic disclosures featured (Pack, 2013, 2014). Harms (2015) similarly discusses the need to maintain self-awareness when dealing with traumatic disclosures as the ability to be self-reflective relies on such awareness.

Once abuse within therapists' own social networks was disclosed, there were often particular flashpoints of stress that affected the therapists' health and well-being. Learning to live with this knowledge that abuse also occurs within one's family of origin, while challenging, enabled Angela, one of the counsellor-participants, to emerge with strategies for dealing with the aftermath following disclosure from family members (Pack, 2013).

## Meso-level: lifestyle and diversity of professional roles

The evolution of an integrated and holistic framework for one's practice as a trauma therapist, achieved by synthesizing a range of theoretical directions, approaches and key concepts on the basis of experiences, personal and professional, became a resource for therapist self-care for the counsellor-participants as it provided a guide for action. Keeping a balance in caseload mix was an important area to reflect upon often to make any necessary adjustments over time. For example, having a mix of trauma and other client work was seen as being an integral part of professional self-care (Pack, 2010a, 2013, 2014).

Being involved in a variety of professional roles and responsibilities was a protective factor enabling the counsellor-participants to continue to practise effectively in the field as trauma therapists. All were involved in a combination of individual therapy, clinical supervision, and teaching, supervising and administering their private practice. Several made these changes quite consciously to sustain their 'freshness for practice' (Angela, counsellor-participant).

To begin with, there was an intensive immersion in trauma therapy and a stepping back to take stock to decide where to place one's energies wisely. Over time, the fear associated with their proximity to trauma seemed to fall away and they described transcending the despair evoked by the traumatic material brought to them by their clients.

Others found increased vigour by changing their lifestyles which involved living closer to nature in rural locations, having a retreat they could escape to away from work, and for some this involved the development of horticultural and agricultural interests. Growing flowers, vegetables, keeping animals and becoming more involved in one's local community were found to be personally and professionally sustaining as careers developed. This sense of connection to the land and neighbours brought them into contact with the wider local community allowing a deeper sense of connection with others with a sense of reciprocity that was missing from their professional lives. While most had been raised with a Christian background, increasingly this connection to the land and to others in local communities was fuelled by a reformulated spirituality. Partly this was a reaction against the patriarchal discourses in organized religion which was related to the use and abuse of power that the counsellor-participants were increasingly aware of through their work as therapists.

## The macro-level: the trauma workforce as a whole – training, professional development and organizational support

On the organizational level of intervention, there are health and safety issues that need to be routinely addressed within organizations working with traumatic disclosures. The risks of engaging with potentially traumatic material need to be explicit during the recruitment of new employees. My research suggests that the risks can be ameliorated if there is sufficient support for workers to draw from a range of theoretical frameworks in an organization that models collaborative approaches and supports collegial behaviour (Pack, 2004, 2013).

These theoretical approaches include but are not limited to trauma-informed, narrative, psychodynamic feminist, systemic theories of practice.

Universities and other providers of counselling and psychotherapy programmes need also to alert students to the potential risks to their psychological health of their involvement in trauma-related helping. Alongside the vicarious traumatization, literature suggesting more positive outcomes needs also to be made available to provide a balance of perspectives from which individuals can select. A range of responses can then inform trainee and prospective workers' views about the work they are undertaking.

Employers have a responsibility for ensuring their workers have access to education about vicarious traumatization. This is particularly important when the focus of the organization is therapy with trauma survivors towards trauma disclosure and recovery. An individualized plan to address vicarious traumatization needs to be developed with the worker, the clinical supervisor and organizational support and, furthermore, to encourage a range of holistic self-care focusing on the physical, psychological, emotional and spiritual dimensions. This organizational focus recommends that clinician self-care, trauma-informed clinical supervision and organizational training are essential to workforce retention, morale and well-being (Berscheit, 2013; Sexton, 1999).

In looking towards the future, this book about trauma therapists' self-care suggests that psychotherapists and other helping professionals need access to a range of options to develop an awareness of vicarious traumatization and resilience in their daily lives and work. It also underlines the importance of trauma therapists sampling and integrating into their practice a range of theoretical approaches that suit what they do in their practice. These approaches, which include narrative, strengths-based and emancipatory frameworks, provide a way for workers to connect with themselves, which naturally fosters effective connections with clients, colleagues and their significant others (Pack, 2004, 2009, 2013). Maintaining relationship is the primary theme of the research on vicarious traumatization. Maintaining connection with self and others protects the counsellor from the fragmenting sense of disjuncture, which is a key experience of trauma-related work. Thus conceptualized, prevention strategies include workers being firmly grounded in theoretical frameworks that provide a context for establishing and maintaining connection on a variety of levels: with the self; with others including clients; with their employing organizations; and with the wider social discourses in which their work is located.

## Conclusion

This book proposes that the ecological systems approach applied to the vicarious traumatization framework produces a holistic, multidimensional approach to understanding therapist self-care on several levels. Such a model attends to the contexts in which vicarious and secondary trauma both develop and impact on trauma therapists. Each level has a central place in the experience of work of therapy and recovery with trauma survivors. There is nothing prescriptive about this, it is simply a matter of awareness and sensitivity to the experience of one's inner self, family and friends, one's clients and to the people one works with in an agency context. In the past ten years, the growth of literature on vicarious traumatization and therapist self-care has expanded and there are now good resources available for the beginning practitioner to become informed about the risks of working with survivors of sexual violence and to build knowledge about what factors support resilience. Some of the core themes in the literature have been outlined, and recommendations for a multilayered approach to intervention made to address vicarious traumatization in work with survivors of sexual violence and trauma from a therapist practitioner perspective (Pack, 2013).

## CONCLUSION AND YOUR SELF-CARE PLAN

Trauma-informed models of clinical supervision are among the most important resources for the worker, and certainly for the reflective practitioner who is either keen to draw on their own sense of awareness when working with clients and to acknowledge their client's healing journey (Cunningham, 2003; Knight, 2006). Relational models of clinical supervision involving specific content related to trauma theory and the application of trauma theory are recommended (Cunningham, 2003; Etherington, 2000, 2009; Knight, 2006).

Ongoing research into the implications of a spiritual dimension for practice is required. How workers see themselves as a resource for survivors of trauma for whom religion and spirituality are important guiding factors in managing their lives is another area requiring further research. This is a thorny issue when abuse survivors may have experienced abuse within organized religion. In relation to this future direction about therapist self-care strategies, we need more information about how we can best inform and educate therapists and other helping professionals who deal with trauma, in the spiritual or intangible aspects of the work of recovery, which is at once intensely personal, and also has a human rights imperative. This is an area where practitioners and service users need, above all, to feel safe and secure and in no way open to coercion or any kind of prescriptive practice.

## Developing your self-care plan

As you finish reading this book, ask what you need to do for your self-care on the micro-, exo-, meso- and macro-levels outlined in this chapter. In each dimension, what do you wish to start doing or what do you need to continue to do to maintain your professional and personal well-being? I suggest using the following checklist as a guide to identify your self-care plan. This is a working document that needs to be time-framed and reviewed regularly. You might wish to do this with a trusted peer or your clinical supervisor as part of your clinical supervision or as a periodic peer review.

## My self-care plan

### The micro-level: individual interventions for self-care

- Think about what is happening to your sleep, appetite and energy which are essential to well-being. Are there any adjustments needed? List three goals in this area.
- In this aspect of self-care, personal therapy needs to be sought if you find that there are issues of your own abuse or trauma intruding into your day-to-day work as a therapist.
- Recurrent dreams or flashbacks involving what clients tell you in their therapy signal the need to attend to this area of self-care, as vicarious traumatization may be impacting.
- Make a note of what needs to be attended to in this area.
- Exploring our identity to know who we are in terms of gender, ethnicity, place, culture and stage of life are other aspects to regularly consider.

### Exo-levels: relationships with significant others

- In this dimension, are those significant others in your personal life getting adequate time with you where you are both physically and emotionally available? If not, what needs to happen?
- Is the work as a trauma therapist affecting your ability to trust and be intimate with your loved one(s)? How so? (Make a note of what you have noticed about your relating to others.)
- What changes (if any) do you wish to make in this area?

### Meso-level: lifestyle and diversity of professional roles

- Is the current balance of your caseload/workload about right or do changes need to be made? List any adjustments that are needed.
- How is your work–life balance currently? Do you wish to diversify into other work/life roles. Make a wish list! List any adjustments/goals/changes that need to be made in this dimension now and for the future. (Aspects to consider in this area include involvement in nature/spirituality/awareness and mindfulness practices.)

### The macro-level: the trauma workforce as a whole – training, professional development and organizational support

- Are you receiving regular clinical supervision that meets your needs as a trauma therapist? What more is needed in this area?
- To what extent are your personal ethics and beliefs aligned or not aligned with your employer's policies and protocols?
- Jot down any thoughts you have about tensions you notice between your personal beliefs and how far these are congruent or not congruent with those of your workplace/ contracting body/group practice.
- Does your workplace provide a comprehensive CISM policy? If not, how could you lobby for what you need with like-minded others/union representation, etc. List goals in this area.
- What other professional development needs do you have? (These might include further personal/professional development, conference attendance, professional association involvement, special interest groups, training in trauma-informed or other theories of practice.)
- In closing, think about what core values are important to you in your practice and check to see that your core values and beliefs can still find expression in the work you do as a therapist. If not, what are the tensions that are impacting in this area of your work/life?
- As you finish this exercise and reading this book, I suggest that you think about what provides replenishment for you in your life more broadly. List three 'next steps' to better align your values with your personal and professional life.

## Closing thoughts

Twenty-two experienced trauma therapists and their significant others contributed to this book hoping their experiences might help and inspire others to learn through their hardships, trials and successes. As they remain engaged in the field of trauma therapy, they continue to find their work sustaining and hopeful within the usual rigours of the work. A large part of their continued hope for their clients and their own lives relies on their matured insights, and the evolution of protective practices. My hope is that this book provides ideas and strategies to continue to evolve relationships, ways of being and lifestyle that support you in your practice, both now and in the future.

# References

Berscheit, K. A. (2013). *A systems view of early interventions for vicarious trauma: Managing secondary trauma stress* (Master's dissertation, St Catherine University). Retrieved from: http://sophia.stkate.edu/msw_papers/151 (accessed 4 March 2016).

Bloemhard, A. (2008). *Spiritual care for self and others.* Coffs Harbour, NSW: Mid North Coast Division of General Practice.

Bronfenbrenner, U. (1994). Ecological models of human development. In *International Encyclopaedia of Education.* Oxford: Elsevier. Retrieved from www.psy.cmu.edu/~siegler/35bronfebrenner94.pdf (accessed 4 March 2016).

Canfield, J. (2005). Secondary traumatization, burnout, and vicarious traumatization. *Smith College Studies in Social Work, 75* (2), 81–101.

Collins, S. and Long, A. (2003). Working with the psychological effects of trauma: Consequences for mental health care workers – a literature review. *Journal of Psychiatric and Mental Health Nursing, 10* (4), 417–24.

Cunningham, M. (2003). Impact of trauma work on social work clinicians: Empirical findings. *Social Work, 48* (4), 451–9.

Etherington, K. (2000). Supervising counsellors who work with survivors of childhood sexual abuse. *Counselling Psychology Quarterly, 13* (4), 377–89.

Etherington, K. (2009). Supervising helpers who work with the trauma of sexual abuse. *British Journal of Guidance and Counselling, 37* (2), 179–94.

Harms, L. (2015). *Understanding trauma and resilience.* London: Palgrave Macmillan.

Harrison, R. L. and Westwood, M. (2009). Preventing vicarious traumatization of mental health therapists: Identifying protective practices. *Psychotherapy Theory, Research, Practice, Training, 46* (2), 203–19.

Hayward, J. (2009). Letter to the editor. *Listener,* 17 October, pp. 6–7.

Herman, J. (1992). *Trauma and recovery.* New York: Basic Books.

Herman, J. (2010). *Trauma and recovery: From domestic abuse to political terror.* London: Pandora.

Johnson, C. N. E. and Hunter, M. (1997). Vicarious traumatization in counsellors working in the New South Wales assault service: An exploratory study. *Work and Stress, 11* (4), 319–28.

Knight, C. (2006). Working with survivors of childhood trauma. *The Clinical Supervisor, 23* (2), 81–105.

Linley, P. A. and Joseph, S. (2007). Therapy work and therapists' positive and negative well-being. *Journal of Social and Clinical Psychology, 26* (3), 385–403.

McCann, C. M., Beddoe, E., McCormick, K., Huggard, P., Kedge, S., Adamson, C. and Huggard, J. (2013). Resilience in the health professions: A review of recent literature. *International Journal of Wellbeing, 3* (1), 60–81.

Marcus, S. and Dubi, M. (2006). The relationship between resilience and compassion fatigue in counsellors. In Walz, G. R., Bleuer, J. C. and Yep, R. K. (Eds). *Vistas: Compelling perspectives on counselling* (pp. 223–5). Alexandria, VA: American Counselling Association.

Medeiros, M. E. and Prochaska, J. O. (1988). Coping strategies that psychotherapists use in working with stressful clients. *Professional Psychology: Research and Practice, 19* (1), 112–14.

Moran, C. C. (2002). Humor as a moderator of compassion fatigue. In Figley, C. R. (Ed.), *Treating compassion fatigue* (pp. 139–54). New York: Brunner-Routledge.

Napier, L. and Fook, J. (Eds). (2001). *Breakthroughs in practice: Theorising critical moments in social work.* London: Whiting & Birch.

O'Halloran, T. M. and Linton, J. M. (2000). Stress on the job: Self-care resources for counselors. *Journal of Mental Health Counseling, 22* (4), 354–65.

Pack, M. (2004). Sexual abuse counsellors' responses to stress and trauma: A social work perspective. *New Zealand Journal of Counselling, 25* (2), 1–17.

Pack, M. (2009). The body as a site of knowing: Sexual abuse therapists' experiences of stress and trauma. *Women's Study Journal, 23* (2), 46–56.

Pack, M. (2010a). Revisions to the therapeutic relationship: A qualitative inquiry into sexual abuse therapists' theories for practice as a mitigating factor in vicarious traumatisation. *Social Work Review: Journal of New Zealand Association of Social Workers, 12* (1), 73–82.

Pack, M. (2010b). Transformation in progress: The effects of trauma on the significant others of sexual abuse therapists. *Qualitative Social Work Research and Practice, 9* (2), 249–65.

Pack, M. (2012). Vicarious traumatisation: An organisational perspective. *Social Work Now: The Practice Journal of Child, Youth and Family, 50,* 14–23.

Pack, M. (2013). Vicarious traumatisation and resilience: An ecological systems approach to sexual abuse counsellors' trauma and stress. *Sexual Abuse in Australia and New Zealand, 5* (2), 69–76.

Pack, M. (2014). Vicarious resilience: A multilayered model of stress and trauma. *Affilia: Journal of Women and Social Work, 29* (1), 18–29.

Pearlman, L. A. and Saakvitne, K. W. (1995). *Trauma and the therapist: Countertransference and vicarious traumatisation in psychotherapy with incest survivors.* New York: Norton.

Pearlman, L. A., Saakvitne, K.W. and staff of the Traumatic Stress Institute. (1996). *Transforming the pain: A workbook on vicarious traumatisation for helping professionals who work with traumatised clients.* New York: Norton.

Reynolds, V. (2011). Resisting burnout with justice-doing. *The International Journal of Narrative Therapy and Community Work, 4,* 27–45.

Sexton, L. (1999). Vicarious traumatisation of counsellors and effects on their workplaces. *British Journal of Guidance and Counselling, 27* (3), 393–403.

Sommer, C. A. (2008). Vicarious traumatisation, trauma-sensitive supervision and counsellor preparation. *Counsellor Education and Supervision, 48* (1), 61–71.

van Heugten, K. (2007). Workplace bullying of social workers. *Aotearoa New Zealand Social Work, 19* (1), 14–24.

van Heugten, K. (2010). Bullying of social workers: Outcomes of a grounded study into impacts and interventions. *British Journal of Social Work, 40* (2), 638–55.

van Heugten, K. (2013). Resilience as an underexplored outcome of workplace bullying. *Qualitative Health Research, 23* (3), 291–301.

White, M. (1995). *Re-authoring lives: Interviews and essays.* Adelaide: Dulwich Centre Publications.

White, M. (1997). *Narratives of therapists' lives.* Adelaide: Dulwich Centre Publications.

## Weblinks and resources on dealing with vicarious traumatization on individual, team and organizational levels

National Child Traumatic Stress Network:

www.nctsn.org/resources/topics/secondary-traumatic-stress

Evidence-based treatments for clients and practitioners, resources, online research, resources for parents and caregivers. Information for the media and for raising public awareness:

www.livingwell.org.au/professionals/confronting-vicarious-trauma

Resources for understanding the neurobiology of trauma, secondary traumatic stress, burnout and vicarious traumatization. Strategies for maintaining health when working with trauma and trauma survivors.

University of Kentucky Center on Trauma and Children:

www.uky.edu/CTAC

'The STSI-OA is an assessment tool that can be used by organizational representatives at any level to evaluate the degree to which their organization is STS-informed, and able to respond to the impact of secondary traumatic stress in the workplace. The STSI-OA identifies specific areas of strength, and opportunities to implement STS-informed policies and practices. The results of this tool can be used as a roadmap for future training and implementation activities in the area of STS and trauma-informed care.'

## CONCLUSION AND YOUR SELF-CARE PLAN

For more information, contact Ginny Sprang, PhD at sprang@uky.edu for training and consulting options. Below is the link to the self-assessment tool aimed at assessing the impact and responsiveness of organizations to secondary traumatic stress: the Secondary Traumatic Stress-Informed Organization Assessment (STSI-OA).

Copyright 2014 Ginny Sprang, Leslie Ross, Kimberly Blackshear, Brian Miller, Cynthia Vrabel, Jacob Ham, James Henry and James Caringi.

www.uky.edu/CTAC/sites/www.uky.edu.CTAC/files/STSI_OA_Final_1.pdf.

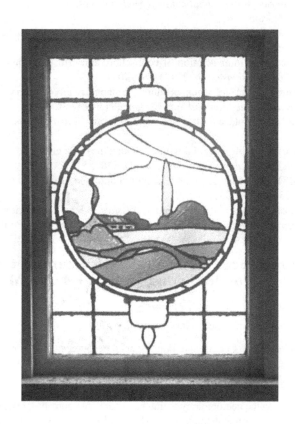

# Index